Hip Replacement

Edited by Carlos Suarez-Ahedo

Published in London, United Kingdom

Hip Replacement
http://dx.doi.org/10.5772/intechopen.98034
Edited by Carlos Suarez-Ahedo

Contributors
Nicolas Padilla-Raygoza, Gilberto Flores-Vargas, Maria De Jesus Gallardo-Luna, Efrain Navarro-Olivos, Francisco J. Magos-Vazquez, Marissa Padilla-Morales, Srino Bharam, Munif Hatem, Hal David Martin, Richard Feng, Livija Šakić, Kata Šakić, Šime Šakić, Jonathan Montomoli, Raffaele Mitri, Emiliano Gamberini, Bijan Dehghani, Neil P. Sheth, Avi Dravid, Praneeth Thota

First published in London, United Kingdom, 2022 by IntechOpen
IntechOpen is the global imprint of INTECHOPEN LIMITED, registered in England and Wales, registration number: 11086078, 5 Princes Gate Court, London, SW7 2QJ, United Kingdom

British Library Cataloguing-in-Publication Data
A catalogue record for this book is available from the British Library

Additional hard and PDF copies can be obtained from orders@intechopen.com

Hip Replacement
Edited by Carlos Suarez-Ahedo
p. cm.
Print ISBN 978-1-80355-759-5
Online ISBN 978-1-80355-760-1
eBook (PDF) ISBN 978-1-80355-761-8

Meet the editor

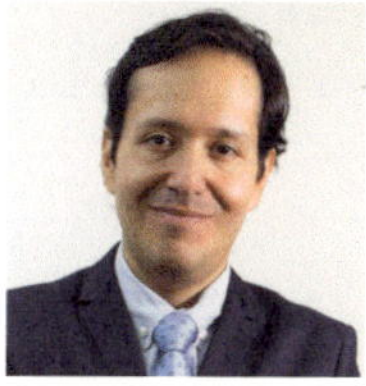

Dr. Suarez-Ahedo is a recognized orthopaedic surgeon with expertise in minimally invasive total hip and total knee replacement, sports medicine, and arthroscopic surgery. He regularly gives lectures and teaches courses for orthopaedic surgeons around the world. He is also the author and co-author of several scientific publications in recognized international journals in the field of sports medicine, arthroscopic surgery, and hip pathology. Dr. Suarez-Ahedo completed his training in Orthopedic Surgery in Mexico City. His subspecialty training includes a fellowship in Articular Surgery, a fellowship in Adult Joint Hip and Knee Reconstruction at the National Rehabilitation Institute of Mexico, and an additional fellowship in Hip Preservation Surgery at the American Hip Institute, Chicago, USA. His professional affiliations include the American Academy of Orthopaedic Surgeons (AAOS), the Arthroscopy Association of North America (AANA), the American Orthopedic Society of Sports Medicine (AOSSM), the International Society for Technology in Arthroplasty (ISTA), The Hip Preservation Society (ISHA), and International Society of Orthopaedic Surgery and Traumatology (SICOT).

Contents

Preface **IX**

Section 1
Anesthesia **1**

Chapter 1 **3**
Regional Anaesthesia for Hip Surgeries
by Livija Šakić, Kata Šakić and Šime Šakić

Chapter 2 **17**
Anesthesia for Hip Replacement
by Jonathan Montomoli, Raffaele Mitri and Emiliano Gamberini

Section 2
Hip Pathology **45**

Chapter 3 **47**
Decision Making in Borderline Cases between Hip Preservation
and Reconstruction Surgery
by Munif Hatem, Richard Feng, Srino Bharam and Hal David Martin

Chapter 4 **71**
Diagnosis of Developmental Dysplasia of the Hip in Newborns
and Infants
*by Nicolás Padilla-Raygoza, Gilberto Flores-Vargas,
María de Jesús Gallardo-Luna, Efraín Navarro-Olivos,
Marissa Padilla-Morales and Francisco J. Magos-Vázquez*

Section 3
Hip Surgery **89**

Chapter 5 **91**
The Direct Anterior Approach: A Comprehensive Guide
for the Learner and Educator
by Bijan Dehghani, Avi Dravid, Praneeth Thota and Neil P. Sheth

Preface

This book provides a concise yet comprehensive introduction to some common hip pathologies and their surgical treatment. It is divided into three sections with short chapters providing a broad overview of anatomy, pathology, and treatment. Selected references are also provided without the claim of being exhaustive and with the aim of stimulating interest and discussion.

Every attempt has been made to narrate the concepts in a simplified manner. Wherever possible illustrations have been used to help the reader to understand the subject. The book is designed for orthopedic surgeons, either in practice or in training, as well as clinicians, radiologists, and physical therapists.

Many people helped make this book. First, I would like to acknowledge IntechOpen and the fantastic team of editors that helped bring this book to fruition. I would also like to especially thank the extraordinary authors who contributed their excellent chapters.

Carlos Suarez-Ahedo
Joints Surgeon (Adults Joint Reconstruction Division,
National Rehabilitation Institute),
Mexico City, Mexico

Section 1

Anesthesia

Chapter 1

Regional Anaesthesia for Hip Surgeries

Livija Šakić, Kata Šakić and Šime Šakić

Abstract

Regional anaesthesia is essential for hip arthroplasty programmes and depends on anaesthesiologist's experienced choice. Good analgesia and the avoidance of post-operative nausea and vomiting are prerequisites for early ambulation and patient compliance with post-operative protocols. Regional anaesthesia, both neuraxial and peripheral nerve blocks, is superior to systemic opioid analgesia at all-time points in the first 3 days following surgery and by avoiding opioids, the risks and incidence of opioid analgesia are removed. Safety of drugs for intrathecal injections and complications from spinal anaesthesia continue to be examined and re-examined in order to improve safety of the technique. Prevention of post-operative cognitive dysfunction and early mobilisation is a key part of the management of patients with hip fractures.

Keywords: regional anaesthesia, analgesia, hip fracture, immune response, hip replacement

1. Introduction

The latest review articles on regional anaesthesia for hip surgery highlight the improvements made in perioperative care combined surgical, anaesthetic and analgesic protocols in order to demonstrate improved perioperative outcomes [1]. The combination of intraoperative spinal anaesthesia with non-opioid adjuvance or low-dose peripheral nerve block (PNB) appears to provide the "ideal" analgesia for hip replacement. The incidence of urine retention requiring catheterisation and post-operative nausea and vomiting is less by avoiding perioperative systemic and intrathecal opioids thus allowing earlier ambulation and discharge. The recent study of Cook et al. confirms that spinal anaesthesia is associated with minimal morbidity of deep vein thrombosis (DVT) and pulmonary embolism (PE) in the majority of cases [2].

2. Sensory innervation of the hip joint

The hip joint is a typical ball-and-socket joint formed by an articulation between the head of the femur and the acetabulum surrounded by a cartilaginous labrum. The entire joint is enveloped by a joint capsule and additionally stabilised by ischiofemoral, iliofemoral and pubofemoral ligament, together with various muscles that either originate in, insert or just pass by this area [3]. Innervation of the hip joint derives from

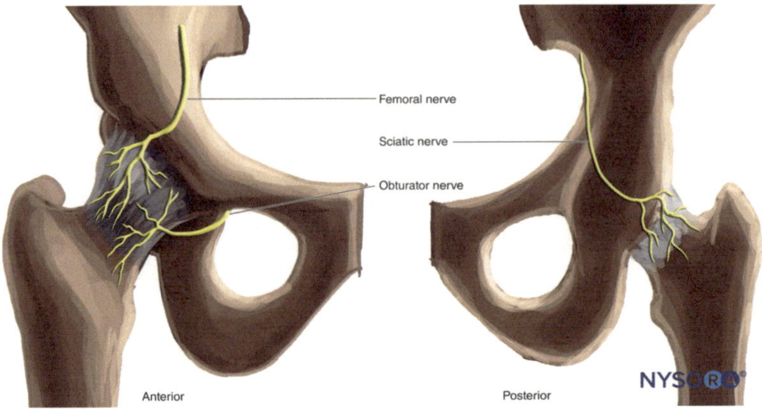

Figure 1.
Sensory innervation of the hip joint.

both lumbar (L1–L4) and sacral (L4–S4) plexuses and the variety of their muscular branches 4. The location of the origin from the main trunk of the nerves providing articular branches to the hip capsule appears to be variable and has only been recorded for the obturator and femoral nerves. There is though substantial discrepancy between studies. According to the studies, most frequent nerve to innervate the hip capsule is the nerve to quadratus femoris muscle followed by the obturator and then the femoral nerve. In general, the course of hip capsule articular branches follows the path of the vessels, but differences in innervation of the hip capsule appear to be present between individuals [4, 5]. Sensory innervation of the hip joint is shown in **Figure 1**.

3. Hip infringements and associated surgeries

Hip fracture implies a fracture of the upper quarter of the femoral bone. Fracture line stretches indifferent directions depending on the force that causes it. According to their anatomical location, hip fractures are classified as intracapsular (IF), which involves the femoral head and neck, and extracapsular (EF), which includes intertrochanteric, trochanteric and subtrochanteric fractures.

Blood loss from an IF at the time of injury is minimal because of the poor vascular supply at the fracture site and tamponade affected by the capsule. Occasionally, fractures without displacement may be treated conventionally, but there is a 30–50% risk of subsequent displacement. Current preference is for all intracapsular fractures without displacement to be treated by internal fixation with multiple screws or a sliding hip screw. Untreated disruption to the capsular blood supply of the head of the femur by a displaced intracapsular fracture can lead to avascular necrosis of the bone, resulting in a painful hip of limited function. Therefore, surgical treatment involves cemented hemiarthroplasty. Blood loss from an EF may exceed one litre; the larger the bone fragments, the greater the blood loss.

In addition, greater periosteal disruption causes EFs to be more painful than an IF. EF is fixed surgically using either a sliding hip screw, (intertrochanteric fractures) or less commonly, a proximal femoral intramedullary nail (subtrochanteric fractures).

In the developed countries, the number of hip replacements has rapidly increased throughout the twenty-one century [6]. This trend is mainly due to the population ageing and according to the lengthening of life expectancy [7].

The rational and the main features of Tissue Sparing Surgery (TSS) concept are maximum respect of anatomy, restoration of joint biomechanics, and removal of degenerated tissues, preserving the healthy ones. So, the prosthesis should just 'integrate' the joint instead of substitute it. The purposes of these techniques are to reduce blood loss, post-operative pain and hospital length of stay while improving recovery and ambulation [8, 9].

Hidden blood loss should not be ignored in patients who underwent hip hemiarthroplasty for displaced femoral neck fractures, as it is a significant portion of total blood loss. A better understanding of HBL after hip hemiarthroplasty may help surgeons improve clinical assessment and ensure patient safety [10].

3.1 Timing of surgery

Recommendations that have been introduced in 1989 by the Royal College of Scientists are that ideally, surgery should be performed within 48 h of hospital admission after hip fracture. In April 2010, new target of 36 h has been accepted in the first place in England and Wales. There are meta-analyses that indicate that delaying surgery beyond 48 h from admission is associated with prolonged in patient stay, increased morbidity (pressure sores, pneumonia, thromboembolic complications) and increased mortality. But, surgery is often delayed because of the need for additional investigation in elderly patients and their preoperative preparation, although there is no evidence to suggest that outcome is improved by delaying surgery to allow preoperative physiological stabilisation. However, the benefits of expedited surgery must be balanced against the risks of certain untreated conditions [11].

4. Central neuraxial anaesthesia in hip trauma and surgery

4.1 Pain in hip trauma and surgery

Pain sensation varies in this type of fractures and surgical reconstructions depending on intensity, quality and duration of pain stimuli involving nociception, inflammation and nerve cell remodelling [12]. Also, nociceptive information strongly influences brain centres for regulating homeostasis. This includes also psychological conditions, such as fear or anxiety that can significantly influence the experience of pain. So, understanding neuroanatomical organisation of central processing of nociceptive information is of great clinical importance.

Proximal femoral fractures are known for most painful injuries and in the elderly, this pain syndrome can even change the cognitive functions. Femoral fractures are usual emergency and characteristically happen in elderly population, which is most vulnerable to the deleterious effects of poorly managed pain, and adverse effects of both drugs and post-operative pain; thus, achieving effective analgesia is particularly difficult because it is necessary to personalise the treatments and, at the same time, the ineffective analgesia may lead to serious complications such as delirium. Untreated severe pain can increase patient's fear and anxiety, lead to aggressive behaviour and disturbance of cognition, and have an unfavourable effect on physiological parameters [11]. These patients jeopardise of perioperative morbidity and mortality, which can be reduced with prompt surgical treatment and punctual quality rehabilitation.

4.2 Neuroendocrine and immune response

Patients with proximal femoral fractures show prolonged adrenocortical response to injury. It is known that elevated cortisol concentrations persist in elderly patients 2 to 3 weeks after injury than in young patients with similar injuries or even more severe. Significantly higher cortisol levels can last up to 8 weeks after injury [12]. The stress hormone cortisol affects the cognitive function, memory and learning, reduces immunity and bone density, and increases body weight, arterial pressure, cholesterol blood levels and heart diseases. Alterations of cognitive status after surgery may present in the form of delirium or, more delicately, as post-operative cognitive dysfunction (POCD). Hyperactivity of the hypothalamo-pituitary-adrenal (HPA) axis with higher cortisol levels is involved in the pathophysiology of delirium [6]; similarly, association between higher plasma cortisol levels and POCD in aged patients following hip fracture surgery occurs [7]. Delirium refers to observable changes in consciousness and attention, whereas POCD may refer to a patient exhibiting significant declines from patient's own baseline level of performance in one or more neuropsychologic domains.

Surgery elicits broad alterations in haemodynamic, endocrine-metabolic and immune responses. The inflammatory response is essential for structural and functional repair of injured tissue, as complement, granulocytes, macrophages and many other mediators are required for appropriate wound healing. Injury, caused by trauma or surgery, is connected with the acute disorder of immunological system, which manifests as increased inclination to infections. The inflammatory response is an important determinant of outcome after major surgery. Perioperative excessive stimulation of the inflammatory and haemostatic systems plays a role in the development of post-operative ileus, ischaemia-reperfusion syndromes (e.g. myocardial infarction), hypercoagulation syndromes (e.g. DVT) and pain. Together, these represent a significant fraction of major post-operative disorders. Regional anaesthesia-administered local anaesthetics prevent or modulate many of these processes.

In the centre of interests, there are the serum-levels of T-helper-1 (Th-1) and T-helper-2 (Th-2) cytokines before and after regional and general anaesthesia and in such a way would like to confirm through the immunological status that the spinal anaesthesia is significantly more favourable for the patient.

Survival depends on the immune system's ability to defend the body against attack from invading pathogens and injury. However, the extent of such a response is of critical importance; deficient responses may result in secondary infections from immunosuppression and excessive responses can be more harmful than the original insult.

Cytokine synthesis and release is an essential component of the innate immune system, but inappropriate, excessive production results in a generalised systemic inflammatory response, which damages distant organs.

The consequences of ageing on the immune system are thought to contribute considerably to morbidity and mortality in the elderly. Tumour necrosis factor-α (TNF-α) and intreleukine-6 (IL-6) concentrations are raised in the elderly, and studies have shown that, in response to surgical trauma, the elderly have a magnified and late inflammatory cytokine response [13].

4.3 Neuromodulation in neuraxial anaesthesia

Regional anaesthesia alone, without surgery, has periodical and minimum effects to immunological system. It is established that various anaesthesiological procedures in the same surgery cause various trend of alteration of cytokine level in serum. Spinal anaesthesia results in less immunosuppression, that is maintains the number of Th-1 cells, thus stimulating the cell immunity. Serious disorder of immunological system may cause complications as there are disorders in wound healing, increased number of infections, non-adequate response to the stress, multi-organic suppression and increased incidence of metastases [14, 15].

Surgery is the best analgesic for hip fractures. It can be performed under the general or regional anaesthesia. There are a great number of studies that analysed and compared the effects of both anaesthetic techniques. There are minimal evidence-based analyses for determining the optimal anaesthetic technique for patients undergoing hip fracture surgery.

Consequently, anaesthesiologists tend to use the technique which they are familiar with half, administering neuraxial anaesthesia and the latter general anaesthesia.

Administration of local anaesthetics was designed to provide intraoperative anaesthesia and post-operative analgesia. However, in recent years it has become clear that regional administered local anaesthetics have benefits far beyond anaesthesia and pain relief; indeed, the technique has significant impact on the outcome of major surgical procedures. A recently published meta-analysis suggests that neuraxial anaesthesia using local anaesthetics decreases overall mortality by approximately one-third, and reduces the odds of DVT by 44%, PE 55%, transfusion requirements by 50%, pneumonia by 39%, and respiratory depression by 59% [16]. There were also reductions in myocardial infarction and renal failure. In addition, epidural anaesthesia using local anaesthetics has been shown to attenuate the endocrine and metabolic response to upper abdominal surgery, to reduce post-operative ileus and to shorten duration of intubation and intensive care stay in patients undergoing abdominal aortic surgery.

Local anaesthetics modulate the inflammatory response *in vivo*. They prevent or reduce inflammatory disorders, such as reperfusion injury in heart. Beneficial effects of local anaesthetic treatment in inflammatory bowel diseases are well documented. In contrast to corticosteroids, which depress the inflammatory response and impact negatively on post-operative outcome, local anaesthetics selectively inhibit only overactive responses of the inflammatory and haemostatic systems without affecting normal function. Local anaesthetics decrease inflammation without increasing the susceptibility to infections and prevent post-operative thrombotic events without increasing bleeding.

Regional anaesthesia-analgesia attenuates perioperative immunosuppression. The hypothesis that patients who receive combined propofol/paravertebral anaesthesia-analgesia (propofol/paravertebral) exhibited reduced levels of protumorigenic cytokines and matrix metalloproteinases (MMPs) and elevated levels of antitumorigenic cytokines compared with patients receiving sevoflurane anaesthesia with opioid analgesia (sevoflurane/opioid). Regional anaesthesia-analgesia for cancer surgery alters a minority of cytokines influential in regulating perioperative cancer immunity. However, any reduction of immunosuppression is less expressed in regional—spinal anaesthesia. Local anaesthetics lidocaine and bupivacaine have influence on a release of IL-1 beta from human lymphocytes *in vitro* reducing chemotaxial and fagocite activity of neutrofiles and inhibits mitogen-induced proliferation of lymphocytes.

Both types of neuraxial anaesthesia, spinal and epidural and general anaesthesia, are associated with impulsive falls in intraoperative blood pressure. Epidural anaesthesia can be used as a sole continuous anaesthetic technique (as a perioperative analgesia and in the same time as an intra-operative anaesthesia) or as a combined spinal-epidural anaesthesia. This regional technique provides excellent analgesia, but may limit early mobilisation after surgery.

Matot et al. in their study from 2003 [17] make a comparison of the analgesic effect of systemic versus continuous epidural analgesia in patients with hip fracture and with high cardiac risk, and came to a conclusion that the incidence of cardiac complications was higher in patients with systemic versus continuous epidural analgesia (11 from 34 patients in systemic analgesia group vs. 2 from 34 patients in group with continuous epidural analgesia). In this study, epidural catheter was placed in early preoperative period due to patients' admission. Few other studies demonstrated that perioperative analgesic management with continuous epidural analgesia started preoperatively reduced the incidence of myocardial ischemia in elderly patients with hip fractures surgery. These result due to sympatholytic effect of local anaesthetic, which in the same time relieves pain and decreases the stress response in perioperative period.

Performing epidural and spinal anaesthesia may be more difficult in elderly patients.

It is often not easy to position the elderly patient appropriately in the lateral position, and frequently, these patients have degenerative changes of the spine. Spinal (subarachnoid) anaesthesia is commonly used, with or without sedation.

Conceptually spinal anaesthesia for hip fracture fixation in elderly patients should be viewed distinctly from spinal anaesthesia for caesarean section in younger patients. Lower doses of intrathecal bupivacaine (< 10 mg) appear to reduce associated hypotension. Co-administration of intrathecal opioids prolongs post-operative analgesia; fentanyl is preferred to morphine or diamorphine, which are associated with greater respiratory and cognitive depression.

Sedation may be provided, but should be used cautiously in the very elderly. Midazolam and propofol are commonly used. Ketamine may be used, theoretically to prevent hypotension, but may be associated with post-operative confusion. Supplemental oxygen should always be provided during spinal anaesthesia.

To achieve general anaesthesia in this group of patients, reduced doses of intravenous induction agents should be administered. Inhalational induction is well tolerated by the elderly and allows for maintenance of spontaneous ventilation. There remains debate about whether mechanical ventilation is preferred to spontaneous ventilation. Paralysis and tracheal intubation are associated with greater physiological derangement than spontaneous ventilation, but proponents argue that mechanical ventilation reduces the risk of perioperative aspiration and allows greater control of arterial carbon dioxide levels. Intraoperative hypoxemia is common, and higher inspired oxygen concentrations may be required.

4.4 Beneficial effects of local anaesthetics

Local anaesthetics for spinal anaesthesia are not only used as drugs to block the sodium channel to provide analgesia and anti-arrhythmic action. Continuous infusion of local anaesthetics has been shown to be the most efficient means to control post-operative pain. Local anaesthetics are the only drugs, which can block almost all the pain pathways involved in post-operative pain. Distribution of local anaesthetics after subarachnoid injection is shown in **Figure 2**. Efficient post-operative pain will not only improve patient's well-being but also accelerate ambulation and decrease the incidence of the post-operative chronic pain syndrome. Interestingly, local anaesthetics also possess anti-inflammatory effects, which may open new indications in different medical settings. Recent research has focused on the use of i.v. local anaesthetics to improve bowel function after surgery or trauma, to protect the central

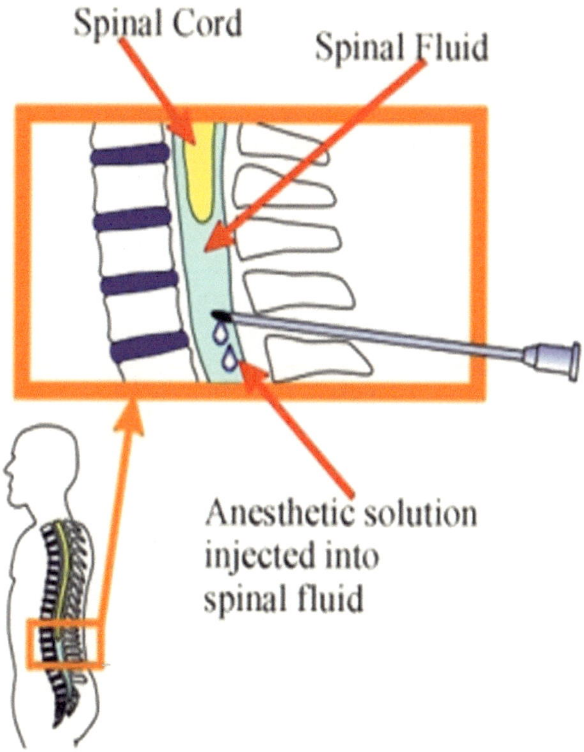

Figure 2.
Application of local anaesthetics after subarachnoid injection.

nervous system, to find new clues of local anaesthetic effect synchronic neuropathic pain and to investigate the long-term effect of anaesthesia/analgesia provided by local anaesthetics on cancer recurrence. There is growing evidence that local anaesthetics have a broad spectrum of indications aside analgesia and anti-arrhythmic effect. Most of them are still insufficiently known and investigated [18].

4.5 Adjuvants in regional anaesthesia

The adjuvants to neuroaxial anaesthesia and peripheral nerve blocks are used in clinical practice: opioids, vasoconstrictors, clonidine, N-methyl-D-aspartate (NMDA) antagonists, γ-aminobutyric acid (GABA) agonists, glucocorticoids, nonsteroidal anti-inflammatory drugs and neostigmine. Analgesia produced by neuraxial opioids alone, or as adjuvants to local anaesthetics, has been demonstrated for acute post-operative pain, obstetric, paediatric and cancer pain [20]. Besides morphine, a number of different opioides and other adjuvants have been introduced to improve the efficacy of neuraxial/regional analgesia, including NMDA antagonists (ketamine, magnesium), GABA agonists (midazolam) and adrenergic agonists (clonidine, adrenaline), COX-inhibitors (ketorolac), acetyl-choline-esterase inhibitor (neostigmine), etc. Any drug given intrathecally rapidly redistributes within the CSF; opioid is detectable in the cisterna magna after lumbar intrathecal administration within 30 min, even with lipophilic drugs like sufentanil.

Glucocorticoids are part of induction of anaesthesia in different clinical protocols achieving much improved analgesia and minimised inflammation with reduced opioid requirements and less adverse events after surgery. Dexamethasone is a long-lasting corticosteroid with effectiveness of 36–54 h [17]. Dexamethasone prolongs sensor and motor blockade with significantly reduced post-operative analgesic requirements, which means it can inhibit phospholipase-A2 and cyclooxygenase-2 expression during inflammation decreasing prostaglandin synthesis [18]. Dexamethasone administered intrathecally affects nuclear transcription in adrenergic receptors [19].

In the study by Bani-hashem et al., intrathecal addition of dexamethasone to bupivacaine for elective orthopaedic surgery on lower limbs significantly prolongs duration of sensory block and decreases opioid requirements in post-operative management. Administration of dexamethasone has the potential to inhibit a patient's endogenous secretion of cortisol. Dexamethasone inhibits corticosterone binding to type II of adrenergic receptors in the pituitary gland passing through the cerebrospinal fluid bound to proteins. Irrelevant of the concentration, dexamethasone has a similar effect on type II of adrenergic receptors. It is possible to resorbs somewhere in the brain without effect on other types of receptors along the HPA axis not depending on the concentration [20]. Single shot of intrathecally administered dexamethasone with levobupivacaine received for surgical treatment of proximal femoral fractures reduces the stress response by decreasing plasma cortisol concentrations with longer lasting analgesic effect with better rehabilitation possibilities [21].

Based on a 2004 Cochrane systematic review of anaesthesia for hip fracture surgery, regional anaesthesia may reduce the incidence of post-operative confusion, the Scottish Intercollegiate Guidelines Network has produced the only recommendation concerning choice of anaesthetic technique, namely that 'spinal, /epidural anaesthesia should be considered for all patients undergoing hip fracture repair, unless contraindicated'. Until such time as evidence is published that confirms regional anaesthesia is superior to general anaesthesia, the Working Party endorses this recommendation. This endorsement is supported by a recent meta-analysis suggesting that regional anaesthesia is the technique of choice (although) the limited evidence available does not permit a definitive conclusion to be drawn with regard to mortality or other outcomes [22].

5. Peripheral nerve blockade for perioperative pain

As explained above, the hip capsule is mainly innervated by the articular branches of the femoral and obturator nerve.

Blockade of the femoral, obturator and lateral cutaneous nerve of the thigh may be sufficient for perioperative analgesia for extracapsular fractures and some intracapsular fractures in trauma surgery.

When considering regional anaesthesia for hip surgery and pain management, there are several different approaches, such as lumbar plexus block/ psoas sheath block, lumbar plexus block/psoas compartment block, lumbar paravertebral block, femoral nerve block, superior gluteal nerve block/sciatic nerve block, spinal and epidural anaesthesia [23–26].

A very reliable method of blocking all three is the psoas compartment block, although this risks a degree of neuraxial blockade and formation of a deep haematoma in recently anticoagulated patients.

Anterior approaches (femoral nerve blockade/fascia iliaca compartment block) do not block all three nerves, but reduce post-operative analgesia requirement, and are more suitable to ultrasound-guided placement and continuous catheter infusions post-operatively. Moreover, in few studies, authors and their colleagues evaluated that especially fascia iliaca compartment block is simple to perform, requires minimal training and also is an effective substitute for conventional treatment of pain in elderly patients with hip fractures. Fascia iliaca compartment block is starting to be used as a routine technique for clinically diagnose hip fracture in the emergency room in various clinical centres in Europe [3].

5.1 Performing the fascia iliaca compartment block (FICB)

The fascia iliaca compartment is a virtual space anteriorly limited by the posterior surface of the fascia iliaca, posteriorly by the iliacus muscle, and is cranially in continuation with the space between quadratus lumborum muscle and its fascia. Three important nerves for hip innervation and sensory innervation of the thigh are located in this space, the femoral nerve, obturator nerve and lateral femoral cutaneous nerve. Lateral femoral cutaneous nerve is a merely sensory nerve originating from the lumbar plexus (L2–L3), emerging from the lateral side of the psoas major muscle and crossing the iliacus muscle obliquely, continuing towards anterior superior iliac spine and passing under the inguinal ligament through the lacuna musculorum. It then divides into anterior branch responsible for sensory innervation of the anterior and lateral thigh as far as the knee, and posterior branch that passes backwards and innervates the skin superior to the greater trochanter down to the middle of the thigh. Additionally, the obturator nerve crosses through the psoas muscle and can be variably blocked by this type of approach. Landmarks for orientation when performing FICB are the anterior superior iliac spine and the pubic tubercle (inguinal ligament). When performing the infra-inguinal approach, this area is divided into thirds, and the injection site is located 1–2 centimetres below the inguinal ligament between the lateral and middle third. It can be performed without ultrasound guidance. When performing without ultrasound guidance, a characteristic '2 pops' are felt that indicate access into the compartment. A study reported an increased frequency of sensory loss in the medial aspect of the thigh when using ultrasound-guided FICB. Similarly, ultrasound guidance increased the frequency of femoral and obturator motor block. Literature also depicts a supra-inguinal ultrasound-guided approach [23]. A supra-inguinal FICB produces a more complete sensory block of the medial, anterior and lateral region of the thigh when compared to infra-inguinal FICB. Likewise, supra-inguinal FICB leads to a more consistent spread in the cranial direction, thus spreading the anaesthetic more consistently towards the lumbar plexus and three targeted nerves. Authors suggest that a sufficient volume to reach femoral nerve, obturator nerve and lateral femoral cutaneous nerve using FICB should be 40 mL. However, the supra-inguinal approach has a superior post-operative analgesic efficacy compared with infra-inguinal approach along with significantly less morphine consumption in the first 24 hours following total hip arthroplasty. **Figure 3a** and **3b** show positioning and longitudinal imaging for ultrasound guided proximal FICB, an in plane approach. Absolute contraindications for this technique are patient's unwillingness to consent to the procedure, known allergy to local anaesthetics, local anaesthetic injection, which has already approached the maximum dosage, previous femoral bypass surgery or close positioning of a graft, local infection at the injection site and relative contraindications are use of anticoagulant therapy with INR >1.5, with need for consideration of recent clopidogrel/high-dose aspirin/low-molecular-weight heparin consumption.

Studies report on paramedics performing FICB on patients with suspected hip fracture at the scene of injury as well [24]. A systematic review on efficacy of prehospital analgesia with FICB for femoral fractures concluded that FICB is suitable for use in the prehospital environment for pain management, with few adverse effects, and can be performed with a high success rate by practitioners of any background. FICB proved to provide superior

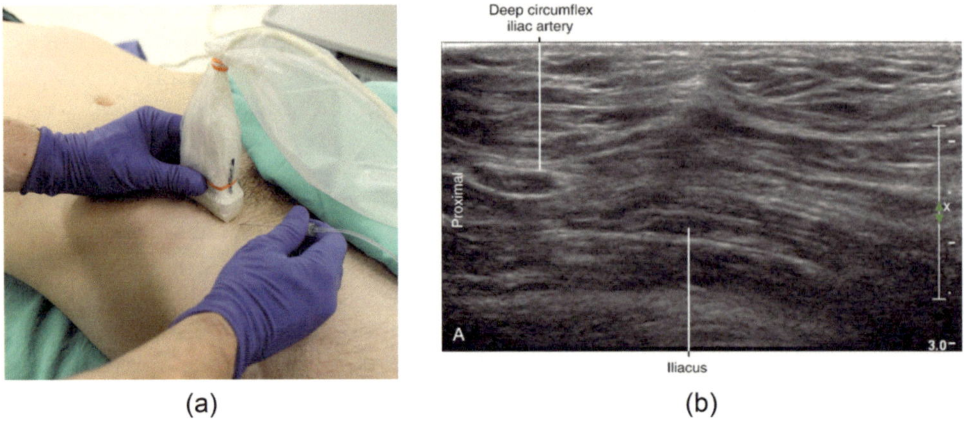

Figure 3.
(a) Positioning for ultrasound guided proximal FICB. In plane approach with longitudinal (coronal) imaging. (3b) Longitudinal imaging for ultrasound guided fascia iliaca block.

analgesia compared to intravenous use of fentanyl before positioning patients for spinal anaesthesia when undergoing surgery for femoral neck fractures of all types. Also, FICB reduced morphine requirement preoperatively for patients with femoral neck fractures, which can be indicated for hip arthroplasty, hip arthroscopy and burn management of the region innervated by nerves blocked by FICB as well. A study reports on reduced morphine consumption after total hip arthroplasty when a longitudinal high-dose supra-inguinal fascia iliaca compartment block was used. Furthermore, continuous femoral block was compared with FICB in patients undergoing hip arthroplasty, and it was concluded that both techniques have equivalent post-operative analgesic efficacy without any difference in functional outcome. Additionally, it was concluded that the fascia iliaca compartment catheter can be placed more quickly than the femoral nerve catheter, but the onset time of sensory and motor blockade is longer when performing the FICB.

5.2 Critical evaluation of quadratus lumborum block

Quadratus lumborum block (QLB), referred to as the 'interfascial plane block', was first described in 2007 as a block of the posterior abdominal wall performed exclusively under ultrasound guidance. It was defined as a variant of a transversus abdominis plane block for a wider analgesia distribution and long-lasting post-operative analgesia. Thoracolumbar fascia (TLF) embeds a thick network of sympathetic neurons and plays an important role in QLB analgesia. However, the true mechanism of analgesia of the QLB is not yet clarified. Local spread of anaesthetics along the TLF is assumed to be accountable for part of the analgesia. Literature describes four different types of QLB depending on the needle tip positioning in relation to QL muscle—anterior, posterior, lateral and intramuscular QLB. In anterior QLB, local anaesthetic is applied in front of the QL muscle, at the level of its attachment to the transverse process of the L4 vertebra. In intramuscular QLB, local anaesthetic is applied directly into QL muscle.

When considering hip surgery and post-operative management, the anterior QLB may play a role in analgesia. It can be performed in a manner that the patient is placed into a lateral position with the needle inserted through the QL in an anteromedial direction. QLB 3—anterior/transmuscular: LA applied in front of the QL muscle, at the level of insertion—transverse process of L4 vertebra.

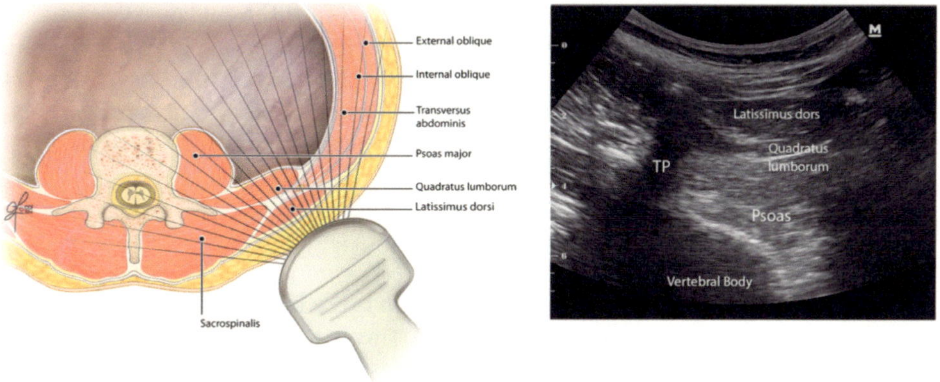

Figure 4.
Scanning technique to identify QL, PM and erector spinae muscles at the level of transverse process (TP) with correaltin ultrasound image on the right.

The local anaesthetic is injected between the QL muscle and psoas major muscle under ultrasound guidance with dosage in the range of 0.2 to 0.4 ml/kg of 0.2 to 0.5% ropivacaine or 0.1 to 0.25% bupivacaine per side is recommended, minimum 15 mL of solution, and one must be aware on highly vascular region [27]. **Figure 4** shows the scanning technique to identify QL, PM and erector spinae muscles at the level of transverse process (TP) with correlating ultrasound image on the right.

Few cases have shown QLB to be beneficial in the management of proximal femoral fractures in high-risk geriatric patients and a patient that underwent hemiarthroplasty after a femoral neck fracture. Few studies also suggest that QLB might provide similar analgesia in comparison with lumbar plexus block for total hip arthroplasty. A role for QLB is in multimodal pain management for hip surgery patients due to its potential for analgesic effectiveness and preservation of muscle strength, which makes it less likely to impair early functional rehabilitation. To summarise, QLB has shown potential for use in hip surgery perioperative pain management, but still lacks sufficient data from prospective studies to be accepted as a reliable treatment approach. Pre- or post-operative peripheral nerve blockade may be used to supplement either general or spinal anaesthesia.

6. Monitoring

Minimum standards for monitoring during the surgery include the continuous presence of the anaesthetist, pulse oximetry, capnography, electrocardiography ECG and non-invasive blood pressure monitoring. Core temperature monitoring should be used routinely. Further monitoring equipment such as invasive blood pressure monitoring, central venous pressure (CVP), cardiac output, bispectral index (BlS) and cerebral oxygen saturation depends of patient's comorbidities.

7. Supplemental pain relief

Regular paracetamol administration should continue throughout the perioperative period. Non-steroidal anti-inflammatory drugs should be used with extreme caution in hip fracture patients and are contraindicated in those with renal dysfunction. Similarly, opioids (and tramadol) should be used with caution in patients with renal dysfunction: oral opioids should be avoided, and both, dose and frequency of intravenous opioids should be reduced (e.g. halved). Codeine should not be administered, as it is constipating, emetic and associated with perioperative cognitive dysfunction.

8. Conclusion

Hip replacement made of experienced surgeon is the best analgesic for hip fractures. Regional anaesthesia is essential for hip arthroplasty programmes depending on anaesthetist's experience and choice. Good analgesia and the avoidance of post-operative nausea and vomiting (PONV) are prerequisites for early ambulation and patient compliance with post-operative protocols. Regional anaesthesia, both neuraxial and peripheral blocks, is superior to systemic opioid analgesia at all-time points in the first 3 days following surgery and by avoiding opioids the risks and incidence of opioid analgesia is removed. Early ambulation is a key part of the management of patients with hip fractures. Safety of drugs for intrathecal injections and complications from spinal anaesthesia continue to be examined and re-examined in order to improve the safety of the technique. More studies will be needed to further understand and improve the clinical use of spinal anaesthesia.

Author details

Livija Šakić[1,2]*, Kata Šakić[2,3] and Šime Šakić[4]

1 Department of Anaesthesiology, Reanimatology and Intensive Medicine, University hospital "Sveti Duh", Zagreb, Croatia

2 Faculty of Dental Medicine and Health Osijek, University of Josip Juraj Strosmayer, Osijek, Croatia

3 School of Medicine, Croatian Catholic University, Zagreb, Croatia

4 Department of Orthopaedic Surgery, School of Medicine, University of Zagreb, Zagreb, Croatia

*Address all correspondence to: mitzilivilla@yahoo.com

References

[1] Macfarlane AJ et al. Does regional anaesthesia improve outcome after total hip arthroplasty? A systematic review. Anaesthesia. 2009;**103**(3):335-345

[2] Cook TM et al. Major complications of central neuraxial block: Report on the Third National Audit Project of the Royal College of anaesthetist. Royal College of Anaesthetists Third National Audit Project. British Journal of Anaesthesia. 2009;**102**(2):179-190

[3] Standring S. Gray's Anatomy International Edition: The Anatomical Basis of Clinical Practice. London: Elsevier Health Sciences; 2015

[4] Halaszynski T, Uskova A. Regional anesthesia for hip surgery. In: Scuderi G, Tria A, editors. Minimally Invasive Surgery in Orthopedics. Cham: Springer; 2016. DOI: 10.1007/978-3-319-15206-6_9-2

[5] Birnbaum K, Prescher A, Hessler S, Heller KD. The sensory innervation of the hip joint--An anatomical study. Surgical and Radiologic Anatomy. 1997;**19**(6):371-375

[6] McPherson K, Gon G, Scott M. International variations in a selected number of surgical procedures. In: OECD Health Working Papers, No. 61. Paris: OECD Publishing; 2013

[7] Pabinger C, Geissler A. Utilization rates of hip arthroplasty in OECD countries. Osteoarthritis and Cartilage. 2014;**22**(6):734-741

[8] Pipino F. Tissue-sparing surgery (TSS) in hip and knee arthroplasty. Journal of Orthopaedics Traumatology. 2006;**7**:33-35

[9] Rossi P, Castoldi F, Rossi R, Caranzano F, Baronetti M, Dettoni F. TSS and traditional surgery in hip and knee replacement. Journal of Orthopaedics Traumatology. 2007;**8**(3):157-120

[10] Kaihang X, Dilixiati A, Rongzhi H, et al. Hidden blood loss after hip hemiarthroplasty using the superPATH approach: A retrospective study. Injury. 2019;**50**(12):2282-2286. DOI: 10.1016/j.injury.2019.10.013

[11] Muhm M, Arend G, Ruffing T, Winkler H. Mortality and quality of life after proximal femur fracture-effect of time until surgery and reasons for delay. European Journal of Trauma and Emergency Surgery. 2013;**39**:267-275

[12] Bisschop PH, de Rooij SE, Zwinderman AH, van Oosten HE, van Munster BC. Cortisol, insulin, and glucose and the risk of delirium in older adults with hip fracture. Journal of the American Geriatrics Society. 2011;**59**:1692-1696

[13] Beloosesky Y, Hendel D, Weiss A, et al. Cytokines and C-reactive protein production in hip-fracture-operated elderly patients. The Journals of Gerontology Series A: Biological Sciences and Medical Sciences. 2007;**62**:420-426

[14] Sakic K, Zura M, Sakic L, Malenica B, Bagatin D, Sturm D. Anaesthetic technique and cytokine response. Periodicum Biologorum. 2011;**113**:151-156

[15] Zura M, Kozmar A, Sakic K, Malenica B, Hrgovic Z. Effect of spinal and general anesthesia on serum concentration of pro-inflammatory and anti-inflammatory cytokines. Immunobiology. 2012;**217**:622-627

[16] Rodgers A, Walker N, Schug S, et al. Reduction of postoperative mortality

and morbidity with epidural or spinal anaesthesia: Results from overview of randomised trials. BMJ. 2000;**321**:1493

[17] Matot I, Oppenheim-Ede A, Ratrot R, et al. Preoperative cardiac events in elderly patients with hip fracture randomized to epidural or conventional analgesia. Anesthesiology. 2003;**98**:156-163

[18] Forget P, De Kock M. Could anaesthesia, analgesia and sympathetic modulation affect neoplasic recurrence after surgery? A systematic review centred over the modulation of natural killer cells activity. Annales Francaises D'anesthesie et de Reanimation. 2009;**28**:751-768

[19] Rathmell JP, Lair TR, Nauman B. The role of intrathecal drugs in the treatment of acute pain. Anesthesia and Analgesia. 2005;**101**:S30-S433

[20] Bani-hashem N, Hassan-nasab B, Pour EA, et al. Addition of intrathecal dexamethasone to bupivacaine for spinal anaesthesia in orthopaedic surgery. Saudi Journal of Anaesthesia. 2011;**5**:382-386

[21] Sakic L, Tonkovic D, Sakic K. Dexamethasone-intrathecal minimiser of simple haemathologic stress biomarkers in hip fracture. Acta Clinica Croatica. 2019;**58**(Suppl 1):9-17. DOI: 10.20471/acc.2019.58.s1.01

[22] Parker MJ, Handol HG, Griffiths R. Anesthesia for hip fracture surgery in adults. Cochrane Database of Systematic Reviews. 2004;**18**:C D0005215

[23] Pepe J, Ausman C, Madhani NB. Ultrasound-guided Fascia Iliaca Compartment Block. In: StatPearls [Internet]. Treasure Island (FL): StatPearls Publishing; 2022. PMID: 30085515

[24] Evans BA, Brown A, Bulger J, Fegan G, Ford S, Guy K, et al. Paramedics' experiences of administering fascia iliaca compartment block to patients in South Wales with suspected hip fracture at the scene of injury: Results of focus groups. BMJ Open. 2019 Feb;**9**(2):e026073

[25] Seidel R, Barbakow E. Surgical treatment of proximal femoral fractures in high-risk geriatric patients under peripheral regional anesthesia : A clinical case series. Anaesthesist. 2019;**68**(2):108-114

[26] Wu CL et al. Efficacy of postoperative patient-controlled and continuous infusion epidural analgesia versus intravenous patient-controlled analgesia withopioids: A meta-analysis. Anesthesiology. 2005;**103**(5):1079-1088

[27] Richman JM, Liu SS, Courpas G, et al. Does continuous peripheral nerve block provide superior pain control to opioids? A meta-analysis. Anesthesia and Analgesia. 2006;**102**:248-257

Chapter 2

Anesthesia for Hip Replacement

Jonathan Montomoli, Raffaele Mitri and Emiliano Gamberini

Abstract

The improvement of surgical and anesthesia techniques has markedly extended the range of patients undergoing hip replacement both in terms of age and comorbidity. Hence, the risk of perioperative complications has increased ranging from hemorrhages, postoperative delirium, incomplete pain control, hypotension, and others. In this regard, a personalized approach from the preoperative evaluation to the choice of the type of anesthesia and the pain control strategy is preferred in order to minimize the risk of complications and accelerate patient's recovering time. In this chapter, we aim to describe different options and propose different possible approaches for the possible scenarios in the light of the existing evidence in the field.

Keywords: general anesthesia, regional anesthesia, hip replacement, complications

1. Introduction

Total hip replacement is one of the most widespread and invasive orthopedic procedures worldwide [1]. In 2007, in the United States, 300,000 surgeries were performed. In the same year, from 50 up to 250 replacements for 100,000 people were carried out in Europe [2]. Total hip replacement has been performed since the 1970s, and upon an appropriate selection of patients, it significantly improves the quality of life by relieving the pain and functional disability experienced by patients with moderate-to-severe arthritis of the hip [2]. Moreover, it is a highly cost-effective procedure [3]. The main indication for surgical treatment remains osteoarthritis, which is particularly disabling among the elderly and obese patients who represent the most prevalent candidates. The other most common indications are:

- primary hip's arthrosis
- rheumatoid arthritis or seronegative autoimmune forms
- femoral epiphysis aseptic osteonecrosis
- post-traumatic arthrosis (results of fractures-dislocations of the femur and/or pelvis)
- secondary arthrosis (associated either with congenital hip dysplasia or with epiphysiolysis or septic arthritis)
- femoral neck's subcapital fractures

Notably, apart from fractures, surgery is, however, recommended only in the event that one of the mentioned pathologies is present in association with severe pain or stiffness that limits daily activities, such as walking, getting up or sitting down, and dressing. Hip prostheses have been performed successfully at all ages, from the young adolescent with juvenile arthritis to the elderly patient with degenerative osteoarthritis [4]. Most of the patients undergoing total hip replacement are between the ages of 50 and 80. However, there is no absolute age or weight limitation for the prosthetic surgery of the hip. The duration of the implants should also be considered; although it has been estimated that roughly 58% of hip replacements will last 25 years [5], their lifespan may markedly vary depending on several factors, being obesity the major cause of a minor longevity of the prosthesis. The indication for surgery is given on the basis of the pain reported by the patient as well as in relation to the degree of disability.

2. Preoperative evaluation

2.1 General considerations

According to the guidelines provided by the European Society of Anesthesia and Intensive Care (ESAIC) for noncardiac surgery, patient's eligibility for surgery should not be based exclusively on strict criteria related to surgery indication, patient's age, weight, and comorbidity, but it is the result of patient's multidimensional assessment with the aim to evaluate the patient's capacity to face and recover from surgery and anesthesia. Such assessment includes the evaluation of the presence and the degree of severity of cardiovascular and respiratory diseases, smoking habit, obstructive sleep apnea syndrome (OSAS), kidney diseases, diabetes, obesity, liver diseases, and alcohol abuse [6]. The assessment of the American Society of Anesthesiologists (ASA) physical status classification system and patient's functional capacity, expressed in terms of metabolic equivalents of task (METS) used to assess energy cost for physical activities or exercise capacity, are two pivotal tools in the evaluation of all patients but may not be sufficient [7, 8]. Interestingly, although the absolute risk for 90-day mortality following total hip replacement is small, a significant increased relative risk has been reported for patients with osteoarthritis younger than 60 and without comorbidity when compared with subject with the same characteristics not undergoing hip surgery [9]. Such increased risk disappears in the long term. On the contrary, there is no increased risk for mortality both in the short and long terms for patients older than 60 and with mild-to-severe comorbidity burden [9]. Such findings indicate that although total hip replacement is a low-risk procedure, it still imposes a risk that becomes most evident in patients with a low baseline mortality risk. The increased relative risk among patients who are young or with a good preoperative prognostic profile may reflect patient-related factors, such as obesity, which may be associated with both the development of osteoarthritis at a young age and an increased procedure-related risk of adverse outcome, including death, as well as system-related factors that might include a lower level of awareness by health professionals toward the prevention, detection, and treatment of thromboembolic complications in patients considered to have a low risk. In addition, relevant comorbidities associated with an increased risk of postoperative mortality, such as liver disease [10], may be undiagnosed in young patients and lead to an inaccurate estimate of the patient's general conditions. Another possible explanation may be the fact that any surgical procedure carries a risk, which, added to a small baseline risk in these patients, results in a high relative mortality.

In conclusion, a systematic preoperative multidimensional assessment of patients undergoing hip replacement should be routinely adopted to detect unrecognized disease and risk factors that may increase the risk associated with the surgical procedures and/or anesthesia techniques above baseline and to propose strategies to reduce this risk.

2.2 Cardiovascular disease

According to the guidelines of the American College of Cardiology (ACA)/American Heart Association (AHA) Task Force, surgical interventions can be classified into three categories according to the risk associated with the procedure itself [11]:

- **High risk**: major surgery in urgency, especially in the elderly, aortic and peripheral arterial vascular surgery, prolonged surgical procedures, and/or associated with significant volume changes.

- **Intermediate risk**: carotid thromboendarterectomy, thoracic and abdominal surgery, head and neck surgery, orthopedic procedures, and prostate surgery.

- **Low risk**: endoscopic procedures, surface surgical procedures, cataract surgery, and breast surgery.

Similarly, patients can be stratified in three categories based on the presence of risk factors for perioperative complications:

- **Major risk factors**: unstable coronary syndromes, acute myocardial infarction (<30 days) with clinical or instrumental evidence of residual ischemia, unstable or disabling angina, heart failure with acute pulmonary edema, severe valvopathy and arrhythmias, atrioventricular block (Mobitz 2 > 2: 1; complete atrioventricular block), and supraventricular arrhythmias with uncontrolled ventricular response.

- **Intermediate risk factors**: stable or controlled angina, previous myocardial infarction, compensated heart failure or previous heart failure, and diabetes mellitus.

- **Minor risk factors**: advanced age, abnormal electrocardiogram (ECG) (left bundle branch block, left ventricular hypertrophy, repolarization's abnormalities, nonsinus rhythm), reduced functional capacity, previous cerebral infarction, and arterial hypertension not controlled by medical therapy or not treated.

The recommendations provided by the AHA/ACC and the ESAIC can be schematically summarized for patients undergoing elective hip replacement as follows: patients with major risk factors require immediate cardiological evaluation, which, in most cases, will lead to myocardial revascularization, valve surgery, or modification of current medical therapy. In this case, the surgery can only be postponed unless it is considered an emergency and, therefore, undelayable. Patients with intermediate risk factors can undergo elective surgery without additional investigations if their functional reserve is at least moderate, and the proposed intervention is at (low or) intermediate risk such as hip replacement. The use of the risk calculator of the American College of Surgeons National Surgical Quality Improvement Program (ACS-NSQIP) is a recommended tool for cardiac perioperative risk stratification. In addition, the assessment of high-sensitivity cardiac troponins in high-risk patients 48 hours before and 72 hours after major surgery is recommended to detect preexisting or postoperative cardiac failure [12]. Therapy with beta blockers should be continued throughout the perioperative period, mostly in patients who have known ischemic heart disease or myocardial ischemia. In patients treated with acetylsalicylic acid, the discontinuation of the therapy should be considered in the perioperative period and should be balanced among the risk of bleeding and the risk of thrombotic complications. For patients undergoing hip replacement, the execution of a baseline electrocardiogram (ECG) in the preoperative period should be mandatory. In the case of patients belonging to the minor-risk class of cardiovascular risk (i.e., elderly patients and patients with a traumatic femur or pelvis fracture) with indication for hip replacement, prolonged monitoring outside the operating room (recovery room/ICU) is strongly recommended, as a good clinical practice to reduce the overall postoperative risk.

2.3 Respiratory disorders

Since chest radiograph rarely alters the perioperative management, it should not be included among the routine investigations. Similarly, spirometry is not recommended as a preoperative routine examination in all patients affected by respiratory problems. On the contrary, patients with obstructive sleep apnea syndrome (OSAS) should be evaluated carefully for potentially difficult airway in the need of ventilatory support or endotracheal intubation. History of previous surgical procedures and referred difficult airway should be investigated especially in patients with diagnosed or suspected OSAS. The use of specific questionnaires to screen for patients with OSAS is recommended when polysomnography (gold standard) is not available. In particularly, among others, the STOP-BANG questionnaire is the most sensitive, specific, and best validated score [13]. Perioperative continuous positive airway pressure (CPAP) must be continued in patients with OSAS to reduce hypoxic events. Moreover, patients with suspected or diagnosed OSAS receiving sedative or general anesthesia during or before surgery should be monitored in the immediate postoperative phase. Of note, stop smoking at least 4 weeks prior to surgery reduces postoperative complications [14].

2.4 Management of antiplatelets/anticoagulant drugs

The perioperative management of anticoagulant therapy is cumbersome due to the complexity of the issue, as well as the simultaneous need to balance the risk of bleeding and the risk of thromboembolic events. On the one hand, surgery should be performed when coagulation is almost normalized to limit the risk of bleeding complications from excessive anticoagulation both during surgery and in the postoperative period. On the other hand, it is necessary to limit as much as possible the interval between the suspension and the restoration of the anticoagulant therapy in order to avoid thromboembolic complications.

A rational approach to the management of anticoagulant therapy should be multidisciplinary and involves the other specialists aiming to carefully evaluate the rationale of the ongoing therapy, the risk of bleeding related to the specific surgical procedure, and the risk of the patient to develop thromboembolic or hemorrhagic events during the complete or suboptimal anticoagulation therapy in the perioperative phase. Taken all together, the final decision should also consider all the therapeutic tools available that are able to modify the coagulation cascade in relation to the specific clinical context [15–18]. Many patients undergoing total hip replacement are on antiplatelet therapy, generally, with low-dose acetylsalicylic acid, ticlopidine, or clopidogrel, more rarely with dipyridamole, indobuphene, or picotamide monohydrate. As for beta blockers, acetylsalicylic acid should be continued in the perioperative period, and its use is associated with a lower incidence of myocardial ischemia in the absence of a substantial increase in surgical bleeding [15]. In general, for medium- and high-risk procedures, clopidogrel should be routinely stopped 7 days before surgery with an exception for patients at high risk of thromboembolic events in whom an interval of 5 days before surgery is recommended and, if available, a platelet function test should be performed to evaluate an adequate platelet function. However, the ACC/AHA Task Force suggests that hip replacement surgery can be safely performed without stopping clopidogrel perioperatively [19]. Ticlopidine is the antiaggregant of choice in patients that are intolerant and/or allergic to acetylsalicylic acid. The antiplatelet effect persists for over 8 days after stopping the drug. The management of ticlopidine therapy in the perioperative period is not codified. For elective hip surgery, it is recommended to discontinue ticlopidine therapy, whereas for emergency procedures, in the case of significant bleeding risk, it would be preferable to perform a platelet transfusion of platelet concentrates [20, 21]. In view of the limited number of relevant publications, it is difficult to release recommendation regarding the perioperative management of antiplatelet therapy with dipyridamole, indobufen, and picotamide. Although some cases of epidural hematoma after locoregional anesthesia have been described in patients receiving acetylsalicylic acid or nonsteroidal anti-inflammatory drugs, the incidence of this complication does not appear to be significantly increased in patients treated with antiplatelet drugs [22, 23]. According to the existing knowledge, locoregional anesthesia is considered suitable for patients on antiplatelet therapy [15, 24]. Similar conclusions may not be drawn for ticlopidine because there is not yet sufficient evidence in the literature. Regarding patients treated with low-molecular-weight heparin (LMWH), heparin should be suspended based on the dosage administered depending on its use as prophylaxis or therapeutic of thromboembolic events. For hip replacement surgery, a 12-hour interval before surgery is recommended when LMWH is used at prophylactic dose. Noteworthy, when a therapeutic dose of enoxaparin (1 mg/kg) is used, a 24-hour interval is recommended. The LMWH can be generally resumed at least 12 hours after hip replacement surgery. The new oral anticoagulants (NAO or DOAC) are a recent class of drugs that act by selectively inhibiting a single coagulation factor, either II or X (**Table 1**), unlike the antivitamin K antagonists (AVK) Warfarin and Acenocoumarol, which act on several factors at the same time (VII, II, IX, and X). DOACs have been introduced

	Dabigatran	**Rivaroxaban**	**Apixaban**	**Endoxaban**
Mechanism of action	**Direct,reversible inhibitor of free anc clot-bound thrombin**	**Direct, reversible inhibitors of free and prothrombinase bound factor Xa**		
Bioavailability	3–7%	80–100%	50%	62%
Protein binding	35%	92–95%	87%	55%
Primary clearance	80% renal	67%renal	56%fecal	50%renal
Tmax	1.5–3 hours	2–3 hours	3–4 hours	1–2 hours
Half-life*	12–14 hours	5–13 hours	12 hours	10–14 hours

Abbreviation: Tmax, time to peak drug concentration after dose.
**Half-life varies with renal function, with increasing half-life, with increased renal impairment.*

Table 1.
Mechanisms of action and characteristics of new oral anticoagulants.

Creatinine clearance	Dabigatran		Apixaban-Rivaroxaban-Endoxaban	
	Low risk surgery	High risk surgery	Low risk surgery	High risk surgery
> = 80 mL/min	> = 24 hours	> = 48 hours	> = 24 hours	> = 48 hours
50-80 mL/min	> = 36 hours	> = 72 hours	> = 24 hours	> = 48 hours
30-50 mL/min	> = 48 hours	> = 96 hours	> = 24 hours	> = 48 hours
15-30 mL/min	Not indicated	Not indicated	> = 36 hours	> = 48 hours

Table 2.
Summary of withdrawal time of new oral anticoagulant stratified by renal clearance and type low versus high risk surgery.

into clinical practice for the prevention of stroke and systemic thromboembolism in patients with atrial fibrillation and for the prevention and treatment of venous thromboembolism. Currently, the DOACs approved by the European Medicines Agency (EMA) on the market are the following:

- Dabigatran etexilate: anti-IIa.
- Rivaroxaban: antiXa.
- Apixaban: antiXa.
- Edoxaban: antiXa.

Table 1 summarizes the mechanisms of action of DOACs. **Table 2** reports the withdrawal times in relation to surgery and renal function.

2.5 Patient blood management and preoperative blood conservation strategies

Anemia is frequent among patients undergoing hip replacement, and its prevalence has been estimated to be up to 25% in patients undergoing hip surgery and markedly increased in the postoperative [25, 26]. The main causes of preoperative anemia are summarized in **Table 3**. Preoperative anemic patients are more likely to receive allogeneic blood transfusions than nonanemic patients. It has been suggested that preoperative anemia and increased blood transfusion rates were independently associated with an increased risk of perioperative adverse outcomes, such as increased postoperative infections, increased hospital length of stay, and increased mortality [27]. Large variability in clinical practice in patient blood management in major orthopedic surgery has been described despite orthopedic surgery is one of the field with the greatest tradition in these programs [26]. Moreover, among patients with anemia, the currently available evidence does not support the use of liberal red blood cell transfusion thresholds based on a 10 g/dL hemoglobin trigger in preference to more restrictive transfusion thresholds based on lower hemoglobin levels or symptoms of anemia in patients undergoing hip fracture surgery [28]. However, criticism on the randomized clinical studies on blood transfusion threshold has been raised regarding the study design and the fact that the decision to transfuse should not be based only on hemoglobin concentrations [29]. Moreover, recent studies using

Insufficient iron intake	Malnutrition, vegetarian diet, vegan diet
Reduced absorption	Gastrectomy,
	Duodenal bypass, bariatric surgery
	H.p. infection, celiac disease
	Atrophic gastritis,
	Inflammatory bowel disease
Chronic blood loss	Gastrointestinal benign and malignant lesions,
	Drugs (salicylates,nonsteroidal anti-inflammatory drugs, corticosteroids)
	Chronic inflammatory bowel diseases
	Polymenorrhea, bladder polyposis
	Congenital hemorrhagic telangiectasia
	Periodic blood donation
Other conditions	Chronic renal failure, heart failure

Table 3.
Main cause of anemia in patients undergoing hip surgery.

sublingual microcirculation monitoring have shown that in critically ill patients with microcirculatory impairment, blood transfusion is able to improve the microcirculation regardless of hemoglobin levels [30, 31]. On the contrary, among patients with normal microcirculation, there are no changes regardless of hemoglobin concentration [30, 31]. Finally, the treatment of preoperative anemia with iron, with or without erythropoietin, and perioperative cell salvage has been reported to decrease the need for blood transfusion [27].

A patient blood management protocol should be adopted in each center and updated regularly. Where feasible, patients programmed for elective surgery should receive a blood count no more than 30 days before surgery, and anemic patients should be referred to the specialist to investigate and treat anemia. The reports of the blood chemistry tests and martial balance are the most common tests for the evaluation of preoperative anemia. The dosage of ferritin, transferrin saturation, and sideremia allow, together with the complete blood count, to make a differential diagnosis of anemia and to personalize the preoperative therapy. **Figure 1** shows a proposed protocol for patient blood management in the preoperative phase.

For the treatment of anemia, there are both intravenous (IV) and oral preparations. Iron sulfate, iron gluconate, and ferric carboxymaltose are the most common in use. Ferric carboxymaltose is usually preferred since it penetrates the bone marrow faster than the other preparation and more rapidly raises the level of serum hemoglobin. This preparation is for intravenous administration only (**Table 4**).

The erythropoiesis stimulating agents (erythropoietin) represents another therapeutic strategy in the patient blood management. The most important indication for the use of erythropoietin perioperatively is the optimization of autologous donation, when indicated or to reduce exposure to allogeneic blood transfusions in adult patients undergoing major elective orthopedic surgery who are at high risk of massive transfusion or for whom a predeposit autologous donation is not available and a blood loss of more than 1000 mL is expected. There are two possible schemes for the use of erythropoietin:

- DIAGRAM 1: Erythropietin 600 U/kg (40.000 U) weekly on days: −21, −14, −7, and on the day of surgery
- DIAGRAM 2: Erythropoietin 300 U/kg (20.000 U) daily from day −10 to day +4 of the surgery.

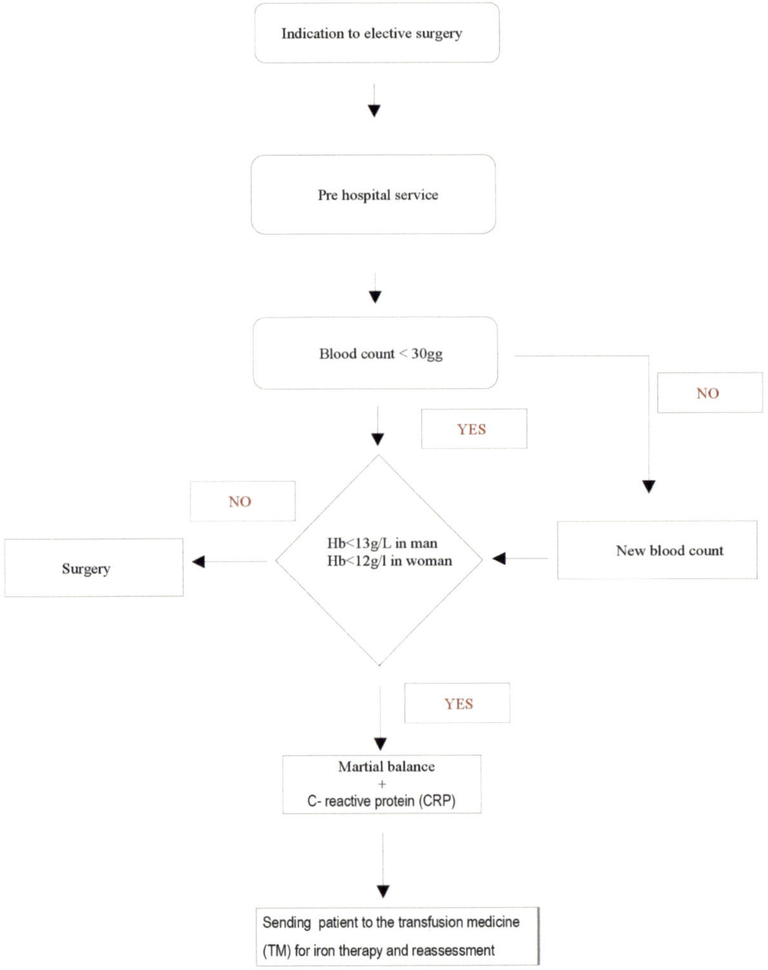

Figure 1.
One of the possible protocols to adopt in the preoperative evaluation of patients undergoing hip surgery inside a patient blood management program.

Hb g/dl	Patients with body weight between 35 Kg and < 70 Kg	Patients with body weight > 70Kg
<10	1500 mg	2000 mg
>/= 10	1000 mg	1500 mg

Table 4.
The cumulative dose of ferric carboxymaltose to be administered on the basis of body weight and hemoglobin levels.

2.6 The geriatric patient

With the aging of the population and the improvement of surgical and anesthesia techniques, the prevalence of elderly patients undergoing hip replacement is growing. In this scenario, the assessment of the functional status become essential, preferably through comprehensive geriatric measures to identify patients at risk and/or to predict postoperative complications. It is strongly recommended to assess the level of independence using validated tools such as *basal and instrumental activities of daily living*. Comorbidities and multiple morbidities become more frequent with aging and are related to increased postoperative morbidity and mortality. It is very useful to assess multiple morbidities using age-adjusted scores, such as the *Charlson comorbidity index* [32, 33]. Elderly patients also take various combinations of drugs (mainly anticholinergics or sedative-hypnotics) increasing the risk of pharmacological interactions with other drugs administered during the hospital admission such as sedative, analgesic, etc. Moreover, these multiple associations often induce unwanted symptoms such as fatigue, anxiety, and delirium, increasing perioperative mortality [34]. It is recommended to consider appropriate perioperative drug adjustments by systematically performing the *BEERS Criteria* for the evaluation of multiple preoperative therapy [35]. Cognitive impairment and depression are common and often underestimated. They can affect patients' ability to understand, thus hindering the full comprehension of the informed consent. The multidimensional geriatric evaluation and teamwork with orthopedics and geriatrics is fundamental. Sensory impairment weakens communication and is associated with postoperative delirium (POD). The assessment of sensory disability should be performed, and the time spent in the perioperative setting without sensory aids should be minimized. Furthermore, malnutrition is relatively common in the elderly, and its impact is often an underestimated factor leading to complications [36]. Malnutrition may also coexist with obesity, further increasing the negative impact on prognosis. Moreover, obesity is associated with an increased risk of kidney damage [37]. The assessment of the nutritional status is very important in order to reduce the duration of hospitalization and shortening the recovery time and must be performed in patients at risk before invasive maneuvers are performed. Finally, as fragility is a known state of extreme vulnerability, frailty assessment in a structured and multimodal way such as the *Fried Score* or the *Edmonton Frailty Scale*, avoiding single surrogate measurements, is also strongly recommended.

2.7 The obese patient

Obesity is associated with metabolic alteration and promote organ failures that should be investigated during the preoperative evaluation. In the preanesthesia evaluation of the obese patients, the evaluation of the airways is among the most important aspects. In addition to the classic Mallampati scale, the evaluation should also include the STOP-BANG questionnaire [13]. Oximetry and/or polysomnography are second-level exams in the overall assessment of OSAS. A neck circumference of at least 43 cm and a high Mallampati score are predictors of both difficult intubation and ventilation. The use of perioperative CPAP is strongly recommended to reduce respiratory complications after surgery.

3. Intraoperative management and anesthesia techniques

3.1 General considerations

There are several validated and safe anesthesia strategies for total hip replacement. In particular, hip replacement represents a challenge for the anesthesiologist who would practice a "tailored" technique, always evaluating the ratio between risk and benefits.

3.2 Monitoring fluid and transfusion administration

All anesthesia techniques may undergo complications. Patient monitoring cannot prevent all adverse events, but there is clear evidence that its application reduces perioperative risks [38, 39]. Total hip replacement surgery can be performed either under general or locoregional anesthesia, and the monitoring must clearly follow standards. All patients should receive electrocardiographic tracing, pulse oximeter, and frequency monitoring. Blood pressure can be reached by noninvasive measurement every 3–5 minutes, otherwise by different interval according to the clinician's opinion [40]. Additional monitoring such as invasive blood pressure, echocardiography, central venous pressure, cardiac output, or other derivative parameters can be adopted in high complexity patients [40, 41]. During general anesthesia and deep sedation, patient's ventilation must be monitored continuously by capnometry in order to confirm a correct ventilation, wherein signs such as respiratory excursions, respiratory rate, and chest auscultation can integrate instrumental monitoring. Although often patients undergoing hip replacement surgery are in spontaneous breathing, capnometry can be used in these cases. Patient's body temperature should also be monitored during anesthesia or sedation in order to minimize patient's discomfort and risk of bleeding. Temperature monitoring and active control systems should be systematically used either in subjects particularly vulnerable to the risk of unintentional hypothermia, such as children and elderly, or during long-lasting procedures with extensive tissue exposure [41]. When neuromuscular blockers are administered, a peripheral stimulator must be available for the monitoring of neuromuscular transmission, and the resumption of normal activity must be measured by the train-of-four (TOF) monitoring. In the last 15 years, specific brain monitoring systems have been introduced into clinical practice. They are based on the analysis of electroencephalogram (EEG) processing or on evoked potentials. However, their use in the routine cannot be considered an integral part of standard monitoring although their use is strongly recommended during total intravenous anesthesia. However, the literature on the possibility of preventing intraoperative awareness using brain monitoring is quite controversial [42, 43]. The use of goal-directed fluid protocols in intermediate-risk patients undergoing hip replacement was studied in few clinical trials. A fluid protocol based on pulse pressure variation (PPV) assessed using continuous invasive arterial pressure measurement seems to be associated with a reduction in postoperative complications and red blood cell transfusion as compared to standard no-protocol treatment [44, 45]. The goal-directed fluid therapy can be guided, in addition to standard monitoring (invasive blood pressure), with devices using pulse contour analysis able to extrapolate the main hemodynamic parameters from the analysis of the pressure wave. Some studies show that by maximizing the stroke volume and the oxygen delivery index, there is a reduction of postoperative complication and a reduction of hospitalization [44, 45]. The rotational thromboelastometer is a point-of-care instrument that studies the viscoelastic properties of whole blood and graphically displays the properties of the clot and its kinetics, from formation to lysis. In particular, it determines the clotting time, the initial time of fibrin formation, the kinetics of fibrin formation and clot development, the strength and stability of the clot, the lysis time, and the platelet function. The thromboelastometer is indicated for the diagnosis, treatment, and monitoring of hemostasis during perioperative bleeding. Among the most frequent causes of bleeding, fibrinolysis is an important one and may be prevented by the infusion of tranexamic acid (TXA) before surgery. Tranexamic acid (TXA) is a synthetic substance, structurally attributable to the amino acid lysine. Tranexamic acid blocks the lysine binding site on the fibrinolytic enzyme plasmin, which is essential for binding plasmin to fibrin. In this way, the fibrinolysis is blocked. TXA reduces blood loss and transfusion administration regardless of the surgical technique. With intravenous preoperative routine use these benefits were seen with both the anterior surgical approach and bilateral hip replacement [46, 47]. The usual dosage of TXA consists of an initial dose of 10–15 mg/kg before surgery that may be followed by an infusion of 1 mg/kg/hour over 4–6 hours or by repeating the initial dose in the postoperative period according to the presence or high risk of bleeding. Recently, local TXA administration in total hip replacement has been investigated, but its use is still controversial. The local application of TXA has been suggested in the consideration of some potential advantages such as easy application, directly affecting the bleeding site, minimizing systemic drug absorption, and, thus, reducing the potential complications of intravenous TXA administration. Local administration should be performed at the end of the surgery, once the fascia is closed, with local injection of 2 g of TXA [48]. In support of this practice, it has been reported that the intravenous use of TXA in total hip replacement significantly reduced blood loss and blood transfusion rates [49]. A recent study shows that the addition of oral TXA for 24 hours postoperatively does not reduce blood loss beyond that achieved with a single 1-g IV perioperative dose alone [50]. An assessment of the risks and benefits in patients is usually recommended. Indeed, in patients with previous thromboembolic events, over 60 years of age, female sex, or undergoing oncological surgery, there is a hypercoagulability's induction and may be not recommended to administer a dose following the initial bolus. As fibrinogen ensures clot formation, the preoperative dosage in patients undergoing elective hip surgery is strongly recommended. Its monitoring during intraoperative bleeding allows for an early supplementation. Fibrinogen's concentrates are the most used molecules. The most recent published guidelines indicate the trigger levels of fibrinogenemia <1.5–2 g/L during massive bleeding. When the indication comes from the monitoring of coagulation carried out through thromboelastographic and metric methods, there is a saving in the use of fibrinogen concentrates. In any case, the use of fibrinogen's concentrate has been shown to have a better cost-benefit ratio. The most common dosage used is 25–50 mg/kg. Intraoperative recovery (RIO) is a blood-saving technique used during intraoperative bleeding. This procedure allows one to reduce the risk of allogeneic transfusions [51]. The blood aspirated and anticoagulated goes into a reservoir, and from there, through filters for microaggregates, it passes into a cell separators bowl to be concentrated by centrifugation, washed with physiological solution and then reinfused. The RIO is indicated with a blood loss of at least 1000 mL or in any case when is expected a blood loss ≥20% of the global volemia, in patients with antibodies which may cause difficulties in transfusion from donor, and in patients who refuse donor blood transfusion. In the case of RIO, the reinfusion consists of red blood cells only. Therefore, in the case of recovery and reinfusion of large volumes, it is important to monitor the platelet count and coagulation [52].

3.3 The importance of normothermia

The relationship between the extent of transfusion support and body temperature is now well established [53, 54]. Hypothermia during surgical procedures is produced by the combination of several factors that participate in the loss of body heat: low temperature in the operating room, administration of unheated fluids, alteration of the mechanisms of thermoregulation induced by anesthesia, and perspiratio insensibilis mainly due to mechanical ventilation. A drop, even moderate, in body temperature is able to modify the physiological mechanisms of hemostasis by altering platelet function and inhibiting the temperature-dependent enzymatic reactions of coagulation [55]. It has been demonstrated that even mild hypothermia (reduction of <1°C in body temperature) can increase blood losses by up to 16%, with a relative increase in the possibility of receiving transfusion therapy (22%) [53, 56]. For these reasons, it is fundamental to ensure the monitoring of the temperature in the operating room and the use of measures aimed at the prevention of hypothermia such as administration of heated fluids, dressing, and active heating.

3.4 Neuraxial strategies

Ideally, all neuraxial techniques for total hip replacement are validated. Therefore, the choice of the specific technique remains at the clinician's discretion. Different techniques can be chosen in relation to the patient, the type of surgical access (e.g., anterior versus posterolateral approaches), and the presumed duration of the surgery. Among the neuraxial procedures, the following are included:

- single-shot spinal anesthesia
- epidural anesthesia
- combined spino-epidural anesthesia
- continuous spinal anesthesia

The single-shot spinal anesthesia is the most used technique. It allows one to keep the patient awake during the surgery, to reduce intraoperative time, and to minimize the administration of intraoperative analgo-sedative drugs, thus allowing for a more rapid discharge from the operating room and reduction of stay [57, 58]. The puncture site is usually at the L3/L4 level, and the most used anesthetic drugs are levobupicavaine or hyperbaric versus isobaric bupivacaine [59]. It is a clinician's choice whether to perform a selective spinal or a total spinal anesthesia for both lower limbs. In any case, the most used dosages vary from 10 to 15 mg for both molecules. With the addition of adjuvant drugs (i.e., clonidine and/or morphine), the duration of anesthesia can be prolonged [60, 61]. Thin needles (27/25 gauge) with Whitacre tip type are less painful on insertion and reduce the number of local complications, such as headache or spinal hematoma [62]. Epidural catheter placement alone is rarely used in this type of surgery. The motor and sensory block necessary for the surgery phase can be reached with high doses of anesthetics. The needle normally used is the Thuoy needle (16/18G) through which a catheter is left in the epidural space. The catheter in place allows the anesthesia to be extended according to the clinician's decision. Managing total surgery time with epidural anesthesia alone may increase the risk of local anesthetic overload toxicity. Combined spino-epidural anesthesia allows for a rapid onset and, if the surgery is prolonged, to continue anesthesia and postoperative analgesia [63, 64]. For elderly patients with fracture surgery, both the general anesthesia and the combined spinal-epidural anesthesia are able to maintain a good anesthesia effect, but the combined spinal-epidural anesthesia is preferable as it may shorten the onset time and it has less impact on the patient's hemodynamic parameters. In addition, combined spinal-epidural anesthesia is associated with lower incidence of complications [63, 64]. Continuous spinal anesthesia is rarely used in hip surgery. It represents a valid alternative to the combined technique as it guarantees an optimal anesthetic plan by reducing the dosage of local anesthetics. On the other hand, it is a procedure that requires an expert team who is familiar with the method [65]. The use of neuraxial anesthesia in routine hip surgery was associated with lower immediate postoperative pain scores, lower intraoperative, and immediate postoperative opioid requirements and may be associated with shorter anesthesia recovery time, without any major adverse events when compared with general anesthesia [66].

3.5 Peripheral nerve and fascial blocks

Nerve blocks consists of the injection of a local anesthetic around a nerve causing pain relief by interrupting transmission of pain signals from the peripheral nerves to the cortex. Nerve blocks for orthopedic procedures have been shown to facilitate the execution of surgery, improve pain control and sleep after surgery, and decrease hospital stay [67, 68]. Nerve blocks may also reduce the need for other analgesic medications, thus limiting associated adverse effects. The hip area is innervated by branches of the lumbar plexus. The hip joint is supplied with femoral and obturator nerves, nerve to quadratus femoris, superior gluteal, and sciatic nerves. The dermatomal supply of the hip joint is typically from spinal nerve roots lumbar-4 to as low as sacral-2. The bony structures of the hip joint are supplied from spinal nerve roots lumbar-3 to sacral-1. It is difficult to achieve complete pain relief of the hip with peripheral nerve blocks [69], and some techniques, such as psoas compartment block, are suggested to be performed by experts [70]. There are many types and techniques for blocking the lumbar plexus nerves following hip replacement:

- Lumbar plexus, or psoas compartment block: a peripheral regional anesthetic technique to block the major nerves of the lumbar plexus (femoral, lateral femoral cutaneous and obturator nerves) in the psoas major muscle [71].

- Femoral nerve block is a safe and widely practiced techniques used for additional local anesthesia and provide postoperative analgesia after hip surgery [72]. Local anesthetic is infiltrated around the femoral nerve, which provides anesthesia to the anterior thigh (femoral nerve) and the medial lower leg (through the saphenous nerve). However, the cephalad spread of the local anesthetic may not be sufficient to block the obturator nerve (medial thigh) and the lateral cutaneous nerve of thigh [73].

- Fascia iliaca compartment block (FICB) is an anterior-thigh regional anesthetic block targeting the lumbar plexus [74]. This block was initially described by Dalens in 1989 for children where sensory blockade of the obturator nerve was believed to be observed. It was believed the local anesthetic spread underneath the iliac fascia proximally toward the lumbosacral plexus [74]. Then, it has been discovered that nearly half of patients do not have a skin component of the obturator nerve and that assessing adductor strength is the only effective way to measure obturator nerve function [75]. The effect of the FICB is similar to the femoral nerve block, but may provide a more reliable method of reaching the femoral lateral cutaneous nerve.

Compared to systemic analgesia alone, it is known that peripheral nerve blocks reduce postoperative pain, acute cognitive impairment, pruritus, and hospitalization [1]. Compared to neuraxial blocks, there is evidence that peripheral nerve blocks reduce pruritus [1]. Severe adverse events with peripheral nerve blocks are fortunately rare, and the use of ultrasound to guide locoregional anesthesia is highly recommended to reduce the risk of unwanted effects (intravenous puncture, local anesthetic systemic toxicity, and intraneural puncture). The ultrasound allows one to recognize the nerve structures in detail, to see in most cases the progression of the needle toward the target nerve structure, and to visualize the diffusion of the local anesthetic [75]. The combined use of the ultrasound system and the electrical nerve stimulator (ENS) increases the success rate in the localization of the nerve and minimizes the possibility of intraneural [76]. The techniques of regional anesthesia may also be useful for the postoperative pain control administering anesthetic drug continuously through a catheter left in the perineural space providing continuous perineural anesthesia/analgesia. A perineural catheter may be left either around the femoral nerve or around the lumbar plexus. The lumbar plexus (psoas compartment) is the first choice for the placement of the continuous perineural anesthesia for total hip replacement [77]. Ultrasound-guided psoas compartment block can be performed with different approaches (i.e., "Lumbar Ultrasound Trident" and "Shamrock technique") [78] and has a lower hemodynamic impact compared to neuraxial techniques especially in elderly patients. Hence, a good anesthetic plan is guaranteed with the possibility to be extended and with a result comparable to other techniques [79]. Finally, an alternative procedure to those already mentioned is the use of the pericapsular nerve group block (PENG block) with local anesthetic infiltration. This technique is still poorly used, but its use is increasing, and it could be hypothesized as an effective and safety anesthesia technique for the total hip surgery [80].

3.6 General anesthesia and multimodal strategies

Sedative or anxiolytic drugs may be used to promote patient comfort and/or facilitate the successful completion of technical procedures such as spinal or locoregional anesthesia. Evidences supporting or the preoperative use of sedative or anxiolytic medication to reduce anxiety and accelerate the achievement of discharge criteria are sparse [81]. Short-acting sedative drugs may be used to facilitate successful completion of technical procedures, but routine administration of sedatives to reduce anxiety preoperatively is not recommended. Among patients undergoing elective primary total hip arthroplasty, general anesthesia has been associated with increased odds of adverse events, prolonged postoperative ventilator use, difficult intubation, stroke, cardiac arrest, other minor adverse events, and blood transfusion [82]. In addition, general anesthesia was associated with mild increases in operative time and postoperative room time [82]. General anesthesia has been previously shown to be associated with pulmonary adverse events following total hip arthroplasty [83].

Compared with neuraxial anesthesia, general anesthesia has been reported to be associated with a higher percentage of intraoperative hypotensive events. This relationship may exist because high-volume surgical centers may be more likely to use spinal anesthesia and may have decreased operative time and room turnover time compared with other centers. In addition, patient extubation likely adds to the postoperative room time. However, despite the significance of these findings, there may be little clinical importance of these minor increases in operating room times [82]. The overall early postoperative mortality in adult patients undergoing hip arthroplasty is low in the absence of risk factors such as severe cardiac hearth failure, chronic obstructive pulmonary disease (COPD), ascites, acute renal failure, and ASA score of 4 or higher. Some studies suggest that there is no association between the type of anesthesia received (general versus regional) and early postoperative mortality rates in patients undergoing hip arthroplasty, regardless of type (total versus partial) [84]. Similarly, other studies show no significant difference between the perioperative blood loss and the occurrence of deep vein thrombosis. However, spinal anesthesia was more advantageous than general anesthesia in terms of the occurrence of nausea and length of stay [85]. In general, large multicenter study on hip and knee replacement are in favor of neuraxial techniques over general anesthesia, and this change in practice has been at the core of established Enhanced Recovery after Surgery (ERAS) guidelines [84, 86]. Large epidemiological studies support the decision toward the choice of central neuraxial anesthesia over general anesthesia showing regional anesthesia being independently associated with better outcomes [87]. However, the claimed superiority of regional anesthesia has been questioned by emerging research. In particular, one single-center randomized clinical trial (RCT) performed in established ERAS centers has questioned whether the reduced cardiopulmonary and thromboembolic complications associated with neuraxial techniques in comparison with general anesthesia are relevant when hip surgery is performed in an ERAS setting where the preoperative optimization and early mobilization of the patient are two important pillars [88]. Harsten et al. compared a modern general anesthesia with a traditional high dose of neuraxial anesthesia (bupivacaine 0.5% 3 mL) and found no clinically relevant differences in functional recovery, hospitalization, urinary complications, and mobilization [88]. General anesthesia may also reduce urinary bladder dysfunction and rare, but potentially severe, neurological complications [89]. Another strategy that may be adopted consists in a multimodal strategy that involved general anesthesia, often conducted with supraglottic airway device, with regional anesthesia most frequently associated with lumbar block. Compared to general anesthesia with endotracheal intubation and combined spinal-epidural anesthesia, general anesthesia with supraglottic airway devices and nerve block had better postoperative analgesic effect and less disturbances on intraoperative hemodynamics and postoperative cognition for elderly patients undergoing intertrochanteric fracture surgeries [90]. Besides the improvement of hemodynamic stability, other advantages of general anesthesia with supraglottic airway device and lumbar plexus and sciatic block (LPSB) included earlier extubation and more rapid weaning from ventilatory support, better control of postoperative pain including longer time to the first analgesic request, and a lower incidence of postoperative complications such as systemic inflammatory response syndrome, pneumonia, sore throat, and hoarseness. In addition, general laryngeal mask anesthesia with LPSB was reported to be associated with a longer postoperative analgesic effect than general anesthesia with endotracheal intubation alone [91]. Another possible option is combining general anesthesia with a supraglottic airway device with fascial block as quadratus lumborum block with or without transversalis fascia plane block) [92, 93]. Preoperative posterior quadratus lumborum block for primary total hip arthroplasty is associated with decreased opioid requirements up to 48 hours, decreased visual analog scale pain scores up to 12 hours, and shorter postanesthesia care unit length of stay [93]. Conversely, other studies did not report benefits in term of opioid postoperative consumption [79]. Therefore, future multicenter RCTs are warranted to further compare the safety issues and potential differences in postoperative morbidity between different anesthetic techniques.

4. Postoperative care

4.1 General considerations

Early mobilization is a key component of hip surgery. Prolonged bed rest causes a series of adverse physiological effects, including increased insulin resistance, myopathy, reduced pulmonary function, impaired tissue oxygenation, and increased risk of thromboembolism. Safe and effective analgesia is a prerequisite to encourage postoperative mobilization. There is substantial evidence that early mobilization facilitates recovery after hip replacement [94].

4.2 Postoperative pain control and acute pain service reality

Postoperative pain is usually a multifactorial acute-on-chronic pain caused by the surgical procedure and the preexisting disease. It is triggered by the response to the trauma of the tissues caused by the surgical act. The control of the postoperative pain is a cornerstone in the postoperative setting and the access to palliative care and pain therapy should be granted. Failure to control postoperative pain has repercussions on the entire system from the patient, by worsening his experience and memories of the already traumatic event, to the hospital structure, by prolonging length of stay, and to the healthcare system, by increasing costs [95]. The postoperative pain therapy should include a preventive approach starting from aiming to a surgical procedure as less invasive as possible such as in case of hip replacement, anterior surgical approach, or robotic surgery [96]. In addition, the so-called preemptive analgesia aims to reduce the initial acute response to pain preventing, or at least limiting, the neuronal modifications associated with windup that consist in a progressively increasing electrical response in the corresponding spinal cord (posterior horn) neurons by repeated stimulation of group C peripheral nerve fibers. Multimodal approach is another preventive technique, with the choice of drugs belonging to different analgesic classes and using techniques of locoregional anesthesia, optimizing analgesia, and minimizing side effects. Similarly, to the anesthesia approach, the pain management after hip replacement should be multimodal, and it must be monitored and managed by an acute pain service (APS). There are different possibilities for postoperative pain control in hip replacement: totally intravenous analgesic infusion, continuous and/or patient-controlled peridural analgesia, and continuous or patient-controlled perineural analgesia; since the first experience of treatment units for acute pain management [97], the benefits of a dedicated and multidisciplinary organization have been reported and accepted, also in terms of cost-effectiveness [98, 99]. Unfortunately, the correct management of postoperative pain is still a challenge in most realities, and APSs are not yet enough diffused. It is possible to differentiate two main APS models: the first is the US model, which consists of anesthesiologist-based comprehensive pain management teams; the second is a nurse-based supervised APS, more diffused in the European countries. A recent Italian study suggests that the creation of the APS model, managed by residents in anesthesia, may represent an alternative between the US model (expensive and difficult to apply in several healthcare systems) and a nurse-based model more frequent in European countries [95].

4.3 Delirium prevention and reduction of length of stay

Postoperative delirium (POD) is one of the most severe complications after surgery, and it is a distressing syndrome both for old surgical patients and their families. It is a complex syndrome that affects 7–65% of patients after hip-fracture surgery [100, 101]. Its social consequences are likely to escalate with a growing old surgical population. The pathogenesis of POD is unclear and probably multifactorial. The most frequent causes are:

- perioperative hypoxemia
- postoperative restorations
- metabolic and electrolyte anomalies
- sleep disturbances
- drugs: opioids, anesthetics, anticholinergics, benzodiazepine, antiparkinsonian drugs
- general anesthesia

The most important predisposing risk factors are:

- elderly
- preexisting cognitive deficits
- multimorbidity
- associated pro-delirious polypharmacy
- insufficient analgesia

Pain is the most common complication after surgical procedures, and it is associated with increased risk of delirium [102]. Conversely, the use of opioids (particularly longer-acting opioids) has also been associated with increased risk of POD [103]. Postoperative mean oxygen saturation at night may also have a role in the development of POD [104]. The mean score of the Mini-Mental State Examination (MMSE) decreased significantly only in patients who received general anesthesia. This suggests that the use of a multimodal opioid-sparing analgesia regime may reduce risk of POD and, therefore, may be considered as a choice especially in patients at high risk for POD. However, there is no consistent evidence about the effects of general anesthesia and regional anesthesia on the incidence of POD following total hip replacement. Even in elderly patients, there was no significant difference in the incidence of cognitive dysfunction 3 months after the use of either general or regional anesthesia [105]. In an RCT among 950 patients aged

65 years and older undergoing hip fracture surgery, regional anesthesia without sedation did not significantly reduce the incidence of POD compared with general anesthesia [91]. The incidence of POD overall was 5.6%. Regardless of the techniques used, patients with POD have been independently associated with adverse clinical and economic outcomes such as death, decreased functional outcome, and cognitive decline, as well as higher cost of care and longer hospitalization. Therefore, it is important to characterize perioperative risk factors related to the incidence of POD and to optimize the quality of care in patients with total hip replacement arthroplasty. Despite the knowledge gaps in delirium pathogenesis, POD may still be preventable with targeted pharmacologic and nonpharmacologic strategies. The first-line preventative interventions for POD are the nonpharmacological interventions. Reorientation is a strategy to help patients get familiarized with the environment and the people. This is done through minimizing staff change and patient transfer, consistent introduction of staff members, access to natural light and time-keeping devices, reminders about the previous events, and future planning. A clinical trial has shown that reorientation alone can reduce the incidence of overt delirium by 40% [106]. Other nonpharmacological interventions include cognitive exercises, vision, sleep and hearing optimization, mobilization, hydration, and nutrition. These interventions are often instituted as a multicomponent care package. The Hospital Elder Life Program (HELP) is a multidisciplinary program designed to prevent cognitive and functional decline in older hospitalized patients, and the focus is on delirium [107]. Nonpharmacologic interventions, such as delirium education programs for medical staff, have led to reductions in delirium duration, hospitalization, and mortality. Antipsychotic drugs are dopamine antagonists and also have varying degrees of affinity to muscarinic, serotonergic, and adrenergic receptors [108]. They are divided into first-generation and second-generation agents, with the first generation (haloperidol) associated with higher risks of psychomotor complications and the second generation associated with higher risks of cardiovascular and metabolic complications. Several studies and meta-analyses have reported that prophylactic administration of second-generation antipsychotics, such as olanzapine and risperidone, may reduce the incidence of postoperative delirium [109]. Because of the risk of complications, the clinical value of antipsychotic prophylaxis is not clear. Pharmacologic ketamine has been found to reduce postoperative inflammation and improve perioperative pain outcomes [110]. In addition, results from a small trial also demonstrated decreased occurrence of delirium and decreased incidence of delayed neurocognitive recovery in cardiac surgery patients who received intraoperative ketamine compared with placebo [110]. Conversely, the PODCAST (Prevention of Delirium and Complications Associated with Surgical Treatments) trial shows that intraoperative ketamine does not prevent delirium. On the contrary, ketamine may increase the risk of adverse perioperative psychoactive experiences [111]. Dexmedetomidine has also been tested in large RCTs in relation to POD and its use is associated with reduction in the composite outcome of delirium, agitation, and confusion [112]. Other drugs have shown some promise as prophylactic agents in noncardiac surgery. These include acetaminophen, ramelteon, gabapentin, statins, clonidine, and melatonin [113].

5. Conclusions

Total hip replacement has been quoted as "the operation of the twentieth century" and one of the most successful and cost-effective procedures in orthopedics. It is usually associated with the high satisfaction of the patients and the improvement of the quality of life following surgery. Great advances in both surgical and anesthesia techniques have allowed us to extend indication for hip replacement to elderly patients with multiple comorbidities. In this regard, the role of the anesthesiologist is fundamental and should follow the patient along his/her entire journey from the preoperative assessment, in order to optimize patient's conditions and plan the best anesthesia technique, to the postoperative recovering to provide an adequate pain control and minimize the risk of preventable complications such as postoperative delirium. A personalized approach has, therefore, become a routinely strategy for anesthesiologists in many specialized centers with all facilities and the necessary know-how. However, there are still several open controversies such as pro and cons related to general versus locoregional anesthesia and the prevention of postoperative complications. Artificial intelligence is among the most promising technology that may further innovate the field of hip replacement in the next years. In particular, machine learning and deep learning methods could markedly improve patient risk stratification and support anesthesiologists in the decision of the best approach to adopt with a specific patient. Such algorithms will need high-quality data to perform with high accuracy and a strong validation process to be trustable but, in return, will provide clinical decision support systems (CDSSs) able to aid physicians in weighing competing healthcare goals and numerous risks by facilitating multiple outcome optimization of outcomes that are too difficult to recognize and navigate on an individual and isolated basis.

This chapter is dedicated to the memory of Tobia Maria.

Conflict of interest

The authors declare no conflict of interest.

Author details

Jonathan Montomoli*, Raffaele Mitri and Emiliano Gamberini
Infermi Hospital, AUSL Romagna, Rimini, Italy

*Address all correspondence to: jonathan.montomoli@auslromagna.it

References

[1] Guay J, Johnson RL, Kopp S. Nerve blocks or no nerve blocks for pain control after elective hip replacement (arthroplasty) surgery in adults. Cochrane Database of Systematic Reviews. 2017 Oct 31;**10**(10):CD011608. DOI: 10.1002/14651858.CD011608.pub2. PMID: 29087547; PMCID: PMC6485776

[2] O'Boyle CA, McGee H, Hickey A, et al. Individual quality of life in patients undergoing hip replacement. The Lancet. 1992;**339**:1088-1091

[3] Faulkner A, Kennedy LG, Baxter K, et al. Effectiveness of hip prostheses in primary total hip replacement: A critical review of evidence and an economic model. Health Technology Assessment. 1998;**2**:1-133

[4] Callaghan JJ, Rosenberg AG, Rubash HE, Clohisy JC, Beaulé PE, Della Valle CJ. The adult hip: hip arthroplasty surgery. Wolters Kluwer Health Adis (ESP). 2015;**1-2**:1624 ISBN: 9781496318473 (Electronic); ISBN: 9781451183696 (Print). [Published: Oct 13 2015]

[5] Evans JT, Evans JP, Walker RW, et al. How long does a hip replacement last? A systematic review and meta-analysis of case series and national registry reports with more than 15 years of follow-up. The Lancet. 2019;**393**:647-654

[6] Lurati BG. Pre-operative evaluation of the adult patient undergoing elective noncardiac surgery: Updated guideline from the European Society of Anaesthesiology Direction and not directives. European Journal of Anaesthesiology. 2018;**35**:405-406

[7] O'Neill F, Carter E, Pink N, Smith I. Routine preoperative tests for elective surgery: summary of updated NICE guidance. BMJ. 2016 Jul 14;**354**:i3292. DOI: 10.1136/bmj.i3292. PMID: 27418436

[8] Fletcher GF, Balady GJ, Amsterdam EA, et al. Exercise standards for testing and training: A statement for healthcare professionals from the American Heart Association. Circulation. 2001;**104**:1694-1740

[9] Pedersen AB, Baron JA, Overgaard S, et al. Short- and long-term mortality following primary total hip replacement for osteoarthritis: A DANISH NATIONWIDE EPIDEMIOLOGICAL STUDY. The Journal of Bone and Joint Surgery British. 2011;**93-B**:172-177

[10] Montomoli J, Erichsen R, Gammelager H, et al. Liver disease and mortality among patients with hip fracture: A population-based cohort study. Clinical Epidemiology. 2018;**10**:991-1000

[11] Fleisher LA, Beckman JA, Brown KA, et al. ACC/AHA 2007 guidelines on perioperative cardiovascular evaluation and Care for Noncardiac Surgery: Executive summary. Journal of the American College of Cardiology. 2007;**50**:1707-1732

[12] Costa MCDBG, Furtado MV, Borges FK, et al. Perioperative troponin screening identifies patients at higher risk for major cardiovascular events in noncardiac surgery. Current Problems in Cardiology. 2021;**46**:100429

[13] Chung F, Abdullah HR, Liao P. STOP-Bang Questionnaire. Chest. 2016;**149**:631-638

[14] Azhar N. Pre-operative optimisation of lung function. Indian Journal of Anaesthesia. 2015;**59**:550

[15] Smith MS, Muir H, Hall R. Perioperative Management of Drug Therapy: Clinical considerations. Drugs. 1996;**51**:238-259

[16] Kearon C, Hirsh J. Management of Anticoagulation before and after elective surgery. The New England Journal of Medicine. 1997;**336**:1506-1511

[17] Wentzien TH, O'Reilly RA, Kearns PJ. Prospective evaluation of anticoagulant reversal with Oral vitamin K1 while continuing warfarin therapy unchanged. Chest. 1998;**114**:1546-1550

[18] Chen AT, Patel M, Douketis JD. Perioperative management of antithrombotic therapy: A case-based narrative review. Internal and Emergency Medicine. 2022 Jan;**17**(1):25-35. DOI: 10.1007/s11739-021-02866-x

[19] Jacob AK, Hurley SP, Loughran SM, et al. Continuing Clopidogrel during elective Total hip and knee arthroplasty: Assessment of bleeding risk and adverse outcomes. The Journal of Arthroplasty. 2014;**29**:325-328

[20] Douketis JD, Spyropoulos AC, Spencer FA, et al. Perioperative Management of Antithrombotic Therapy. Chest. 2012;**141**:e326S-e350S

[21] Aaron SH, Jagan R, John RH. Perioperative platelet transfusions. Anesthesiology. 2021;**134**:471-479. DOI: 10.1097/ALN.0000000000003670

[22] Horlocker TT, Wedel DJ, Schroeder DR, et al. Preoperative antiplatelet therapy does not increase the risk of spinal hematoma associated with regional anesthesia. Anesthesia & Analgesia. 1995;**80**:303-309

[23] Kietaibl S, Ferrandis R, Godier A, et al. Regional anaesthesia in patients on antithrombotic drugs: Joint ESAIC/ESRA guidelines. European Journal of Anaesthesiology. 2022;**39**: 100-132

[24] Muscatelli SR, Charters MA, Hallstrom BR. Time for an Update? A look at current guidelines for venous thromboembolism prophylaxis after hip and knee arthroplasty and hip fracture. Arthroplasty Today. 2021;**10**:105-107

[25] Lasocki S, Krauspe R, von Heymann C, et al. PREPARE: The prevalence of perioperative anaemia and need for patient blood management in elective orthopaedic surgery: A multicentre, observational study. European Journal of Anaesthesiology. 2015;**32**:160-167

[26] Abad-Motos A, Ripollés-Melchor J, Jericó C, et al. Patient Blood Management en artroplastia primaria de cadera y rodilla. Encuesta entre los investigadores del estudio POWER.2. Revista Española de Anestesiología y Reanimación. 2020;**67**:237-244

[27] Spahn DR. Anemia and patient blood Management in hip and Knee Surgery. Anesthesiology. 2010;**113**:482-495

[28] Brunskill SJ, Millette SL, Shokoohi A, Pulford EC, Doree C, Murphy MF, Stanworth S. Red blood cell transfusion for people undergoing hip fracture surgery. Cochrane Database Systematic Reviews. 21 Apr 2015;(4):CD009699. DOI: 10.1002/14651858.CD009699.pub2. PMID: 25897628

[29] Vincent J-L. Transfusion thresholds: The dangers of guidelines based on randomized controlled trials. Intensive Care Medicine. 2020;**46**:714-716

[30] Sakr Y, Chierego M, Piagnerelli M, et al. Microvascular response to red blood cell transfusion in patients with severe sepsis. Critical Care Medicine. 2007;**35**:1639-1644

[31] Scheuzger J, Zehnder A, Meier V, Yeginsoy D, Flükiger J, Siegemund M. Sublingual microcirculation does not reflect red blood cell transfusion thresholds in the intensive care unit-a prospective observational study in the intensive care unit. Crit Care. 2020 Jan 17;**24**(1):18. DOI: 10.1186/s13054-020-2728-7. PMID: 31952555; PMCID: PMC6969438

[32] Charlson ME, Pompei P, Ales KL, et al. A new method of classifying prognostic comorbidity in longitudinal studies: Development and validation. Journal of Chronic Diseases. 1987;**40**:373-383

[33] Brusselaers N, Lagergren J. The Charlson comorbidity index in registry-based research: Which version to use? Methods of Information in Medicine. 2017;**56**:401-406

[34] Anderson BJ, Liu M, Cui X, et al. Adverse outcomes associated with inpatient Administration of Beers List Medications Following Total Knee Replacement. Clinical Therapeutics. 2020;**42**:592-604.e1

[35] By the 2019 American Geriatrics Society Beers Criteria® Update Expert Panel. American Geriatrics Society 2019 Updated AGS Beers Criteria® for Potentially Inappropriate Medication Use in Older Adults. Journal of the American Geriatrics Society. Apr 2019;**67**(4):674-694. DOI: 10.1111/jgs.15767. Epub 2019 Jan 29. PMID: 30693946

[36] Meyer M, Kappenschneider T, Grifka J, et al. Risikomanagement in der orthopädischen Chirurgie: Stratifizierung und Adjustierung patientenindividueller Risikofaktoren. Orthopade. 2022;**51**:81-90

[37] Hennrikus M, Hennrikus WP, Lehman E, Skolka M, Hennrikus E. The obesity paradox and orthopedic surgery. Medicine (Baltimore). 2021 Aug 20;**100**(33):e26936. DOI: 10.1097/MD.0000000000026936. PMID: 34414951; PMCID: PMC8376337

[38] Fowler AJ. A review of recent advances in perioperative patient safety. Annals of Medicine and Surgery (Lond). 2013 Nov 14;**2**(1):10-14. DOI: 10.1016/S2049-0801(13)70020-7. PMID: 26977290; PMCID: PMC4326122

[39] Lienhart A, Auroy Y, Péquignot F, et al. Survey of anesthesia-related mortality in France. Anesthesiology. 2006;**105**:1087-1097

[40] Meng L, Yu W, Wang T, Zhang L, Heerdt PM, Gelb AW. Blood Pressure Targets in Perioperative Care. Hypertension. 2018 Oct;**72**(4):806-817. DOI: 10.1161/HYPERTENSIONAHA.118.11688. PMID: 30354725

[41] Buhre W, Rossaint R. Perioperative management and monitoring in anaesthesia. The Lancet. 2003;**362**: 1839-1846

[42] American Society of Anesthesiologists Task Force on Intraoperative Awareness. Practice advisory for intraoperative awareness and brain function monitoring: a report by the american society of anesthesiologists task force on intraoperative awareness. Anesthesiology. 2006 Apr;**104**(4):847-64. DOI: 10.1097/00000542-200604000-00031. PMID: 16571982

[43] Kertai MD, Whitlock EL, Avidan MS. Brain monitoring with electroencephalography and the electroencephalogram-derived Bispectral index during cardiac surgery. Anesthesia & Analgesia. 2012;**114**:533-546

[44] Benes J, Haidingerova L, Pouska J, et al. Fluid management guided by a

continuous non-invasive arterial pressure device is associated with decreased postoperative morbidity after total knee and hip replacement. BMC Anesthesiology. 2015;**15**:148

[45] Cecconi M, Fasano N, Langiano N, et al. Goal-directed haemodynamic therapy during elective total hip arthroplasty under regional anaesthesia. Critical Care. 2011;**15**:R132

[46] Zha G-C, Zhu X-R, Wang L, et al. Tranexamic acid reduces blood loss in primary total hip arthroplasty performed using the direct anterior approach: A one-center retrospective observational study. Journal of Orthopaedics and Traumatology. 2022;**23**:12

[47] Sarpong NO, Chiu Y-F, Rodriguez JA, et al. Simultaneous bilateral Total hip arthroplasty with contemporary blood management is associated with a low risk of allogeneic blood transfusion. The Journal of Arthroplasty. 2022;**37**:544-548

[48] Gilbody J, Dhotar HS, Perruccio AV, et al. Topical tranexamic acid reduces transfusion rates in Total hip and knee arthroplasty. The Journal of Arthroplasty. 2014;**29**:681-684

[49] Örs Ç, Çaylak R. The efficacy, safety, and cost-effectives of combined administration of intravenous and local tranexamic acid in the management of patients undergoing primary Total hip arthroplasty: A prospective, blinded and randomized clinical study. Acta Orthopaedica et Traumatologica Turcica. 2021;**55**:422-427

[50] Magill P, Hill JC, Bryce L, et al. Oral tranexamic acid for an additional 24 hours postoperatively versus a single preoperative intravenous dose for reducing blood loss in total hip arthroplasty: Results of a randomized controlled trial (TRAC-24). Bone Joint Journal. 2021;**103-B**:1197-1205

[51] Laranjeira H, Coimbra C, Fernandes N, et al. Postoperative recovery of blood in patients undergoing total knee or hip arthroplasty. Acta Médica Portuguesa. 2013;**26**:511-516

[52] Carless PA, Henry DA, Moxey AJ, O'Connell D, Brown T, Fergusson DA. Cell salvage for minimising perioperative allogeneic blood transfusion. Cochrane Database Systematic Reviews. 2010 Apr 14;**2010**(4):CD001888. DOI: 10.1002/14651858.CD001888.pub4. PMID: 20393932; PMCID: PMC4163967

[53] Pan P, Song K, Yao Y, et al. The impact of intraoperative hypothermia on blood loss and allogenic blood transfusion in Total knee and hip arthroplasty: A retrospective study. BioMed Research International. 2020;**2020**:1-6

[54] Rajagopalan S, Mascha E, Na J, et al. The effects of mild perioperative hypothermia on blood loss and transfusion requirement. Anesthesiology. 2008;**108**:71-77

[55] Ruetzler K, Kurz A. Consequences of perioperative hypothermia. Handbook of Clinical Neurology. 2018;**157**:687-697. DOI: 10.1016/B978-0-444-64074-1.00041-0. PMID: 30459033

[56] Sessler DI. Perioperative thermoregulation and heat balance. The Lancet. 2016;**387**:2655-2664

[57] Imbelloni LE, Beato L. Comparação entre raquianestesia, bloqueio combinado raqui-peridural e raquianestesia contínua para cirurgias de quadril em pacientes idosos: estudo retrospectivo. Revista Brasileira de Anestesiologia. 2002;**52**:316-325

[58] Koc M, Sacan O, Gamli M, et al. Retrospective evaluation of anesthesia

techniques for hip replacement operations. Turkish Journal of Anesthesiology & Reanimation. 2014;**42**:133-139

[59] Glaser C, Marhofer P, Zimpfer G, et al. Levobupivacaine versus racemic bupivacaine for spinal anesthesia. Anesthesia & Analgesia. 2002;**94**:194-198

[60] Crespo S, Dangelser G, Haller G. Intrathecal clonidine as an adjuvant for neuraxial anaesthesia during caesarean delivery: A systematic review and meta-analysis of randomised trials. International Journal of Obstetric Anesthesia. 2017;**32**:64-76

[61] Vitalis CF, Mung'ayi, Thikra S. A randomised controlled trial comparing the effect of adjuvant intrathecal 2 mg midazolam to 20 micrograms fentanyl on postoperative pain for patients undergoing lower limb orthopaedic surgery under spinal anaesthesia. African Health Sciences. 2016;**16**:282

[62] Campbell DC, Douglas MJ, Pavy TJG, et al. Comparison of the 25-gauge Whitacre with the 24-gauge Sprotte spinal needle for elective caesarean section: Cost implications. Canadian Journal of Anaesthesia. 1993;**40**:1131-1135

[63] Zhong H, Wang Y, Wang Y, Wang B. Comparison of the effect and clinical value in general anesthesia and combined spinal-epidural anesthesia in elderly patients undergoing hip arthroplasty. Experimental and Therapeutic Medicine. 2019 Jun;**17**(6):4421-4426. DOI: 10.3892/etm.2019.7465. Epub 2019 Apr 3. PMID: 31086576; PMCID: PMC6489064

[64] Cazeneuve JF, Berlemont D, Pouilly A. Value of combined spinal and epidural anesthesia in the management of peroperative analgesia in prosthetic surgery of the lower limb. Prospective study of 68 cases. Revue de Chirurgie Orthopédique et Réparatrice de l'Appareil Moteur. 1996;**82**:705-708

[65] Imbelloni LE, Gouveia MA, Cordeiro JA. Continuous spinal anesthesia versus combined spinal epidural block for major orthopedic surgery: Prospective randomized study. São Paulo Medical Journal. 2009;**127**:7-11

[66] Turner EHG, Whalen CJ, Beilfuss MA, et al. Neuraxial anesthesia is associated with decreased pain scores and post-anesthesia care unit opioid requirement compared with general anesthesia in hip arthroscopy. Arthroscopy: The Journal of Arthroscopic & Related Surgery. 2021;**37**:139-146

[67] Ilfeld BM, Gearen PF, Enneking FK, et al. Total knee arthroplasty as an overnight-stay procedure using continuous femoral nerve blocks at home: A prospective feasibility study. Anesthesia & Analgesia. 2006;**102**:87-90

[68] Ilfeld B, Gearen P, Enneking F, et al. Total hip arthroplasty as an overnight-stay procedure using an ambulatory continuous psoas compartment nerve block: A prospective feasibility study. Regional Anesthesia and Pain Medicine. 2006;**31**:113-118

[69] de Visme V, Picart F, Le Jouan R, et al. Combined lumbar and sacral plexus block compared with plain bupivacaine spinal anesthesia for hip fractures in the elderly. Regional Anesthesia and Pain Medicine. 2000;**25**:158-162

[70] The Regional Anesthesiology and Acute Pain Medicine Fellowship Directors Group. Guidelines for fellowship training in regional anesthesiology and acute pain medicine: Third edition, 2014. Regional Anesthesia and Pain Medicine. 2015;**40**:213-217

[71] Capdevila X, Biboulet P, Morau D, et al. Continuous three-in-one block for postoperative pain after lower limb orthopedic surgery: Where do the catheters go? Anesthesia & Analgesia. 2002;**94**:1001-1006

[72] Cauhèpe C, Oliver M, Colombani R, et al. The '3-in-1' block: Myth or reality? Annales Françaises d'Anesthèsie et de Rèanimation. 1989;**8**:376-378

[73] Marhofer P, Oismüller C, Faryniak B, et al. Three-in-one blocks with Ropivacaine: Evaluation of sensory onset time and quality of sensory block. Anesthesia & Analgesia. 2000;**90**:125-128

[74] Dalens B. Regional anesthesia in children. Anesthesia and Analgesia. 1989;**68**:654-672

[75] Bouaziz H, Vial F, Jochum D, et al. An evaluation of the cutaneous distribution after obturator nerve block. Anesthesia & Analgesia. 2002;**94**:445-449

[76] Dufour E, Quennesson P, Van Robais AL, et al. Combined ultrasound and Neurostimulation guidance for popliteal sciatic nerve block: A prospective, randomized comparison with Neurostimulation alone. Anesthesia & Analgesia. 2008;**106**:1553-1558

[77] de Leeuw MA, Zuurmond WWA, Perez RSGM. The psoas compartment block for hip surgery: The past, present, and future. Anesthesiology Research and Practice. 2011;**2011**:1-6

[78] Behr AU, Vasques F. The thumb-up: a different view of the Shamrock lumbar plexus block. Minerva Anestesiol. 2018 Dec;**84**(12):1422-1423. DOI: 10.23736/S0375-9393.18.12933-6. Epub 2018 May 28. PMID: 29808976

[79] Aksoy M, Dostbil A, Ince I, et al. Continuous spinal anaesthesia versus ultrasound-guided combined psoas compartment-sciatic nerve block for hip replacement surgery in elderly high-risk patients: A prospective randomised study. BMC Anesthesiology. 2014;**14**:99

[80] Sandri M, Blasi A, De Blasi RA. PENG block and LIA as a possible anesthesia technique for total hip arthroplasty. Journal of Anesthesia. 2020;**34**:472-475

[81] Møiniche S, Kehlet H, Dahl JB. A qualitative and quantitative systematic review of preemptive analgesia for postoperative pain relief. Anesthesiology. 2002;**96**:725-741

[82] Basques BA, Toy JO, Bohl DD, et al. General compared with spinal anesthesia for Total hip arthroplasty. The Journal of Bone and Joint Surgery. 2015;**97**:455-461

[83] Helwani MA, Avidan MS, Ben Abdallah A, et al. Effects of regional versus general anesthesia on outcomes after Total hip arthroplasty: A retrospective propensity-matched cohort study. The Journal of Bone and Joint Surgery-American. 2015;**97**:186-193

[84] Khan IA, Noman R, Markatia N, Castro G, Rodriguez de la Vega P, Ruiz-Pelaez J. Comparing the effects of general versus regional anesthesia on postoperative mortality in total and partial hip arthroplasty. Cureus. 2021 Jan 3;**13**(1):e12462. DOI: 10.7759/cureus.12462. PMID: 33552779; PMCID: PMC7854317

[85] Pu X, Sun J. General anesthesia vs spinal anesthesia for patients undergoing total-hip arthroplasty: A meta-analysis. Medicine. 2019;**98**:e14925

[86] McDonald DA, Siegmeth R, Deakin AH, et al. An enhanced recovery

programme for primary total knee arthroplasty in the United Kingdom — Follow up at one year. The Knee. 2012;**19**:525-529

[87] Memtsoudis SG, Sun X, Chiu Y-L, et al. Perioperative comparative effectiveness of anesthetic technique in orthopedic patients. Anesthesiology. 2013;**118**:1046-1058

[88] Harsten A, Kehlet H, Toksvig-Larsen S. Recovery after total intravenous general anaesthesia or spinal anaesthesia for total knee arthroplasty: A randomized trial † †this article is accompanied by editorial IV. British Journal of Anaesthesia. 2013;**111**:391-399

[89] Kehlet H, Aasvang EK. Regional or general anesthesia for fast-track hip and knee replacement - what is the evidence? F1000Res. 2015;**4**: F1000 Faculty Rev:1449

[90] Liu Y, Su M, Li W, et al. Comparison of general anesthesia with endotracheal intubation, combined spinal-epidural anesthesia, and general anesthesia with laryngeal mask airway and nerve block for intertrochanteric fracture surgeries in elderly patients: A retrospective cohort study. BMC Anesthesiology. 2019;**19**:230

[91] Chen W, Guo N, Wang S, et al. General laryngeal mask airway anesthesia with lumbar plexus and sciatic block provides better outcomes than general anesthesia and endotracheal intubation in elderly patients undergoing hip surgery. Archives of Gerontology and Geriatrics. 2018;**78**:227-232

[92] Vasques F, Stecco C, Mitri R, De Caro R, Fusco P, Behr AU. Blocking around the transversalis fascia: behind the scene. Minerva Anestesiol. 2019 Jan;**85**(1):15-20. DOI: 10.23736/S0375-9393.18.12479-5. Epub 2018 Mar 27. PMID: 29589417

[93] Kukreja P, MacBeth L, Potter W, et al. Posterior quadratus lumborum block for primary total hip arthroplasty analgesia: A comparative study. Einstein (São Paulo). 2019;**17**:eAO4905

[94] Soffin EM, YaDeau JT. Enhanced recovery after surgery for primary hip and knee arthroplasty: A review of the evidence. British Journal of Anaesthesia. 2016;**117**:iii62-iii72

[95] Borracci T, Prencipe D, Masotti A, et al. The experience of setting up a resident-managed acute pain service: A descriptive study. BMC Anesthesiology. 2015;**16**:14

[96] Fontalis A, Epinette J-A, Thaler M, et al. Advances and innovations in total hip arthroplasty. SICOT-Journal. 2021;**7**:26

[97] Ready LB, Oden R, Chadwick HS, et al. Development of an anesthesiology-based postoperative pain management service. Anesthesiology. 1988;**68**:100-106

[98] Bardiau FM, Braeckman MM, Seidel L, et al. Effectiveness of an acute pain service inception in a general hospital. Journal of Clinical Anesthesia. 1999;**11**:583-589

[99] Stadler M, Schlander M, Braeckman M, et al. A cost-utility and cost-effectiveness analysis of an acute pain service. Journal of Clinical Anesthesia. 2004;**16**:159-167

[100] Dasgupta M, Dumbrell AC. Preoperative risk assessment for delirium after noncardiac surgery: A systematic review: RISK ASSESSMENT FOR DELIRIUM AFTER NONCARDIAC SURGERY. Journal of the American Geriatrics Society. 2006;**54**:1578-1589

[101] Bin Abd Razak HR, Yung WYA. Postoperative delirium in patients undergoing Total joint arthroplasty:

A systematic review. The Journal of Arthroplasty. 2015;**30**:1414-1417

[102] Bilge EU, Kaya M, Senel GO, et al. The incidence of delirium at the postoperative intensive care unit in adult patients. Turkish Journal of Anaesthesiology & Reanimation. 2015;**43**:232-239

[103] Weinstein SM, Poultsides L, Baaklini LR, et al. Postoperative delirium in total knee and hip arthroplasty patients: A study of perioperative modifiable risk factors. British Journal of Anaesthesia. 2018;**120**:999-1008

[104] Rosenberg J, Kehlet H. Postoperative mental confusion--association with postoperative hypoxemia. Surgery. 1993;**114**:76-81

[105] Rasmussen LS, Johnson T, Kuipers HM, et al. Does anaesthesia cause postoperative cognitive dysfunction? A randomised study of regional versus general anaesthesia in 438 elderly patients. Acta Anaesthesiologica Scandinavica. 2003;**47**:260-266

[106] Colombo R, Corona A, Praga F, et al. A reorientation strategy for reducing delirium in the critically ill. Results of an interventional study. Minerva Anestesiologica. 2012;**78**:1026-1033

[107] Singler K, Thomas C. HELP – Hospital Elder Life Program – ein multimodales Interventionsprogramm zur Delirprävention bei älteren Patienten. Internist. 2017;**58**:125-131

[108] Farah A. Atypicality of atypical antipsychotics. Prim Care Companion Journal of Clinical Psychiatry. 2005;**7**:268-274

[109] Wu Y-C, Tseng P-T, Tu Y-K, et al. Association of Delirium Response and Safety of pharmacological interventions for the management and prevention of delirium: A network meta-analysis. JAMA Psychiatry. 2019;**76**:526

[110] Martocchia A, Curto M, Comite F, et al. The prevention and treatment of delirium in elderly patients following hip fracture surgery. Recent Patents on CNS Drug Discovery. 2015;**10**:55-64

[111] Avidan MS, Maybrier HR, Abdallah AB, et al. Intraoperative ketamine for prevention of postoperative delirium or pain after major surgery in older adults: An international, multicentre, double-blind, randomised clinical trial. The Lancet. 2017;**390**:267-275

[112] Su X, Meng Z-T, Wu X-H, et al. Dexmedetomidine for prevention of delirium in elderly patients after non-cardiac surgery: A randomised, double-blind, placebo-controlled trial. The Lancet. 2016;**388**:1893-1902

[113] Asleson DR, Chiu AW. Melatonin for delirium prevention in acute medically ill, and perioperative geriatric patients. Aging Medicine. 2020;**3**:132-137

Section 2

Hip Pathology

Chapter 3

Decision Making in Borderline Cases between Hip Preservation and Reconstruction Surgery

Munif Hatem, Richard Feng, Srino Bharam and Hal David Martin

Abstract

The hip joint is the center of human body movement. An optimal hip function is critical for general health, mental health and well-being. A frequent dilemma in orthopedic practice is what to recommend to a patient with hip pain who is neither the ideal candidate for hip preservation surgery nor for total hip arthroplasty. What are the factors to be considered when deciding between a hip preservation or replacement surgery? This chapter aims to help orthopedic surgeons to decide between hip preservation or total hip arthroplasty as the primary surgery for borderline cases. Chondral damage, age, acetabular dysplasia, femoral torsion abnormality, lumbar spine disease, patient expectation, abnormalities in more than one hip layer, comorbidities, and psycho-social determinants are the main factors to be considered on decision-making for hip surgery. Conservative management, hip arthroscopy, hip osteotomy, and total hip arthroplasty can also be seen as a continuum of treatment.

Keywords: hip preservation surgery, surgery indication, hip arthroplasty, hip arthroscopy, hip osteotomy

1. Introduction

Orthopedic surgeons treating patients with hip disorders often see borderline cases between hip preservation surgery and total hip arthroplasty (THA). This scenario is becoming more frequent following the advancements in hip preservation surgery techniques in the last 3 decades.

Hip preservation surgery and THA may also be seen as a continuum of treatment. This approach is utilized in many clinical disorders in different medical fields. When treating heart failure, for example, cardiologists will try less invasive clinical and surgical approaches before proceeding with a heart transplant. As in prior times of technological advancement, hip preservation surgery and THA have progressed allowing for a better understanding of the complex hip-spine-pelvic-CORE anatomy and biomechanics of each of the five hip layers: the osteochondral, capsulolabral, musculotendinous, neurovascular, and kinematic chain, the interpretation of which is dependent on a comprehensive history and physical examination, with triplanar

• Degree of chondral disease
• Patient age
• Acetabular and femoral abnormalities
  • Acetabular dysplasia
  • Femoral torsion and acetabular version abnormalities
  • Ischiofemoral impingement
• Presence of low back pain
• Other factors:
  • Patient expectations
  • Abnormalities in additional hip layers
  • Contra-lateral hip disease
  • Profession and physical activities
  • Chronicity of pain
  • Family support
  • Commitment to rehabilitation
  • Opioid use
  • Comorbidities and psychological factors
  • Physician-related factors

Table 1.
Factors to take into consideration to decide between hip preservation versus reconstruction surgery.

imaging assessment. Osseous conditions of the hip affect other hip layers in a cascading fashion.

The decision for borderline cases between preservation and reconstruction is complex, and the physician is intuitively considering multiple factors to be shared with patient. Frequently, a patient prefers the risk of a failed hip arthroscopy than the potential complications of a total hip arthroplasty. Therefore, the role of the orthopedic surgeon is to be well informed and make the decision with his patient. Similar cases based on imaging findings may require different approaches (conservative, hip preservation or THA) based on patient's expectations.

The goal of this chapter is to organize factors and evidence to help the reader on the decision-making process for borderline cases between preservation and THA. This chapter does not aim to say what is right and what is wrong, it aims to help the reader to make the best decision for the patient based on the patient expectations. As an important reminder, the orthopedic surgeon is not required to make the decision in a single appointment, and repeat assessments are often the best way to define the most appropriate treatment approach for each patient. Repeat visits also helps to build relationship with patients, which is a key component in outcomes. The elements to be discussed in the current chapter are organized as in **Table 1**.

2. Degree of chondral damage

The degree of chondral damage is the first element to consider in borderline cases between hip preservation and reconstruction surgery. The results of hip preservation surgery are inferior in individuals with more advanced chondral disease [1]. The degree of chondral damage observed at the time of surgery is associated with risk of conversion to THA after hip arthroscopy. McCarthy et al. reported the likelihood of THA at a mean follow-up of 13 years after hip arthroscopy according to the cartilage disease observed arthroscopically [2]. Femoral head chondral damage was the strongest risk factor for conversion to THA. Hips with Outerbridge Grades III-IV disease at the femoral head were 58 times more likely to require conversion to THA when compared to Outerbridge Grades 0–2 [2]. Hips with acetabular cartilage disease Grade II-IV were 20 times more likely to require conversion to THA when compared to Outerbridge Grades 0–1. For patients who underwent THA, McCarthy et al. reported an average time of 4.8 years between the hip arthroscopy and THA [2]. Horisberger et al. reported the rate of conversion to THA in 20 patients with generalized degenerative changes at the hip joint observed during arthroscopy [3]. From 20 patients, 50% had undergone or planned to undergo a THA at a mean follow-up of 3 years. The mean time between the hip arthroscopy and THA was 1.4 years [3].

Preoperative imaging studies are helpful to estimate the risk of conversion to THA after hip preservation surgery [3, 4]. Hip joint space measurements on standing and supine pelvic radiographs have been shown to be equivalent by Bessa et al. [5]. Philippon et al. described that hips with joint space <2 mm at pre-operative radiograph were 39 times more likely to progress to a THA than those with ≥2 mm of joint space [6]. Larson et al. reported that 82% of the individuals with pre-operative joint space narrowing (>50% joint space narrowing compared to contra-lateral normal hip or ≤ 2 mm of joint space) failed to improve above 70 points on Harris Hip Score or underwent THA at a mean follow-up of 27 months. Zimmerer et al. studied the 11-year hip survivorship in 112 patients after primary hip arthroscopy according to the pre-operative Tönnis grade [4]. Conversion to THA was observed in 54% of the hips with Tönnis 2 or 3. In contrast, 14% of hips with no or minimal osteoarthritic changes on radiographs (Tönnis 0 or 1) underwent a THA following the primary hip arthroscopy at a mean follow-up of 11 years [4]. Modern techniques of labral repair may affect previously reported outcomes and need further studies.

Despite the usefulness of pre-operative imaging to estimate the degree of chondral damage, conventional radiographs and magnetic resonance imaging (MRI) underestimate the severity of chondral disease in 3 out of 4 patients with marked generalized chondral lesions [3]. For hips with more than 2 mm of joint space or Tönnis grade 0 and 1, Rosinsky et al. reported that narrower joint space was not correlated with intraoperative cartilage damage (**Figure 1**) [7]. The authors mentioned that narrower joint space (above 2 mm) may be an anatomic variant and cannot predict actual intraoperative cartilage damage [7].

The frequent conversion to THA after hip preservation surgery in hips with advanced acetabular chondral damage at long term does not mean patients cannot benefit from hip preservation at short and mid-term. Peters et al. reported improved Harris hip scores from an average of 68 preoperatively to 91 at a mean follow-up of 26 months after open treatment for femoroacetabular impingement in 39 hips with Outerbridge grade 4 acetabular chondral damage [8]. Despite the good clinical outcomes, the authors described radiographic progression of osteoarthritis in 43% of the hips with Outerbridge grade 4 acetabular chondral damage [8]. The above paper reinforces that functional and clinical assessment are essential in association to radiographic evaluation when making clinical decisions for patients with degenerative changes at the hip. The effects of limited hip mobility on the lumbar spine and pelvis also need to be considered and will be discussed later in this chapter (**Figure 2**).

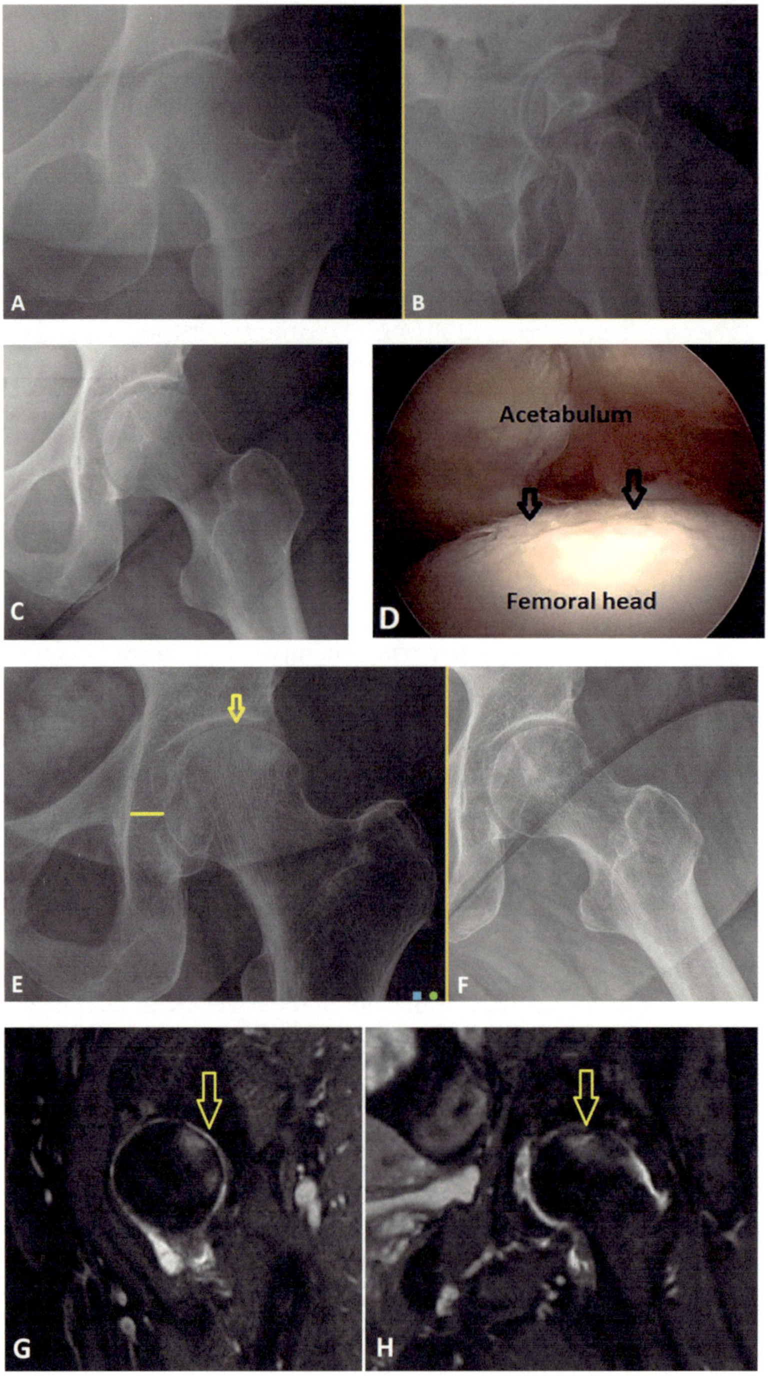

Figure 1.
Imaging of a 67-year-old patient who was recommended total hip arthroplasty 1 year after hip arthroscopy. Femoral head chondral damage observed arthroscopically, despite preserved joint space pre-operatively. Figures A, B and C) radiographs demonstrating joint congruency and preserved joint space; D) arthroscopic image demonstrating the chondral damage at the femoral head (arrows); E and F) 10 months post-operative radiographs demonstrating lateral migration of the femoral head (yellow line) and subtle narrowing of the joint space; G and H) 10 months post-operative magnetic resonance imaging demonstrating the chondral damage with subchondral edema, not observed in the pre-operative MRI.

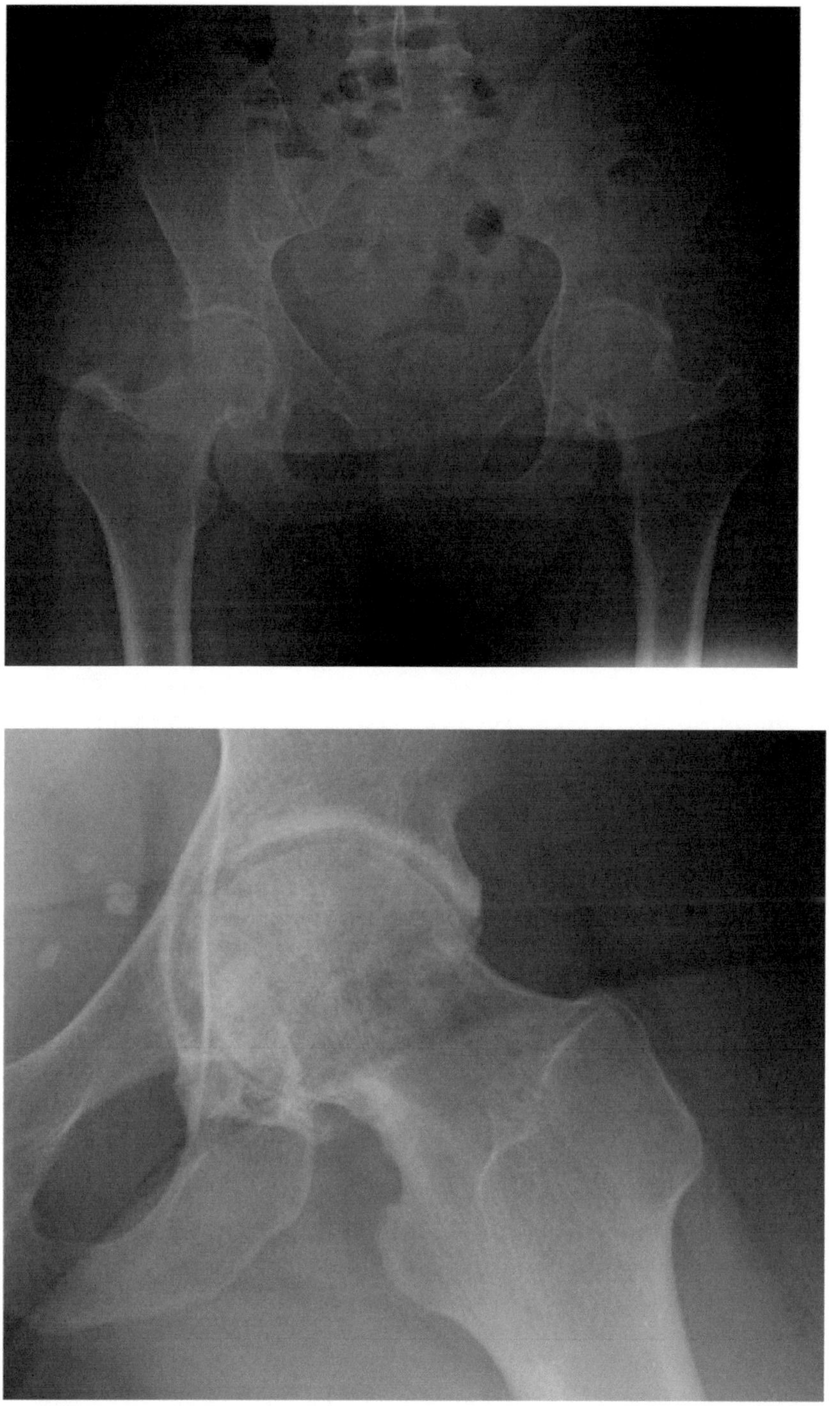

Figure 2.
Anteroposterior and lateral radiographs of a 53 years-old female with advanced left hip osteoarthritis and four years of conservative management including anti-inflammatory medication and intra-articular injection with corticosteroid. Modified Harris hip scores for the left hip is 93.5 out of 100.1. In contrast to the very satisfactory right Harris hip score, the Oswestry lumbar disability score has worsened from 8 to 16% in one year. This patient illustrates the importance of clinical assessment in association to imaging studies, as well as the effects of decreased hip mobility at the lumbar spine, when making clinical decisions for patients with hip diseases.

Hips with cam femoroacetabular impingement and advanced chondral damage often progress with anterosuperior migration of the femoral head to the cartilage defect. This finding has been recognized as a landmark for progressive osteoarthritic changes [9]. The anterosuperior migration of the femoral head is usually not evident on the anteroposterior or lateral radiographs. False profile of Lequesne radiographs and magnetic resonance are fundamental to identify the anterosuperior migration of the femoral head to the cartilage defect. The authors of the current chapter believe the migration of femoral head is a turning point on the progression of femoroacetabular impingement to be considered when recommending a hip preservation surgery. Hips with cam morphology and anterosuperior migration of the femoral head to the chondral defect are under the risk of further instability and rapid progression of osteoarthritis if undergoing a hip preservation surgery.

3. Age

The incidence of hip arthroscopy for older adults has grown exponentially along the last 2 decades. An increase of 280% in incidence of hip arthroscopy has been observed in the United States from 2005 to 2014 in the Medicare population, with 8100 primary hip arthroscopies performed [10].

Two variables are considered when studying hip arthroscopy results in older patients: 1) Improvement on functional scores; 2) Conversion rate to THA. A randomized controlled trial by Martin et al. compared hip arthroscopy and physical therapy versus physical therapy alone for patients older than 40 years with limited osteoarthritis (Tönnis grades 0–2) [11]. Arthroscopic acetabular labral repair with postoperative physical therapy led to better outcomes than physical therapy alone [11]. Martin et al. also reported a cross-over rate of 64% for patients from the non-surgical group to the hip arthroscopy group after 14 weeks, i.e., 64% of patients needed surgery after unsuccessful physical therapy [11]. Horner et al., in a systematic review published in 2017, concluded that patients over 40 years-old undergoing hip arthroscopy including femoral osteochondroplasty and labral repair presented clinically significant improvements in most research studies, whereas labral debridement did not produce clinically significant improvements postoperatively [12]. In a clinical scenario, the clinician should consider the difference in "normal" values for functional hip scores according to the age when making treatment recommendations or comparing results. Sharfman et al. compared the patient-reported outcomes measures among 3 different age groups for non-symptomatic individuals: <40 years, 40 to 60 years, and > 60 years [13]. The iHOT, mHHS, HOS-ADL, and HOS-Sport of these asymptomatic respondents all decreased in an age-dependent manner: iHOT (<40, 94.1; 40–60, 92.4; >60, 87.0), mHHS (<40, 94.8; 40–60, 91.3; >60, 89.1), HOS-ADL (<40, 98.4; 40–60, 95.0; >60, 90.9), and HOS-Sport (<40, 95.7; 40–60, 82.9; >60, 72.9) [13]. The authors stressed the importance of comparing a patient's outcome scores with the age-normalized scores to establish an accurate reference frame with which to interpret outcomes [13]. In advancing age, the hip function grows in importance to maintain mental and general health.

The conversion rate to THA after hip arthroscopy is another factor to consider when recommending hip arthroscopy to older patients. According to Malik et al., the native hip was preserved at 2 years after surgery in 81.5% Medicare patients who underwent primary hip arthroscopy between 2005 and 2014 [10]. Patients >65 years had a 20% THA rate versus a 15% THA rate for below 65 years of age at 2 years after the hip arthroscopy [10]. Horner et al., in a systematic review, reported a rate of conversion to THA of 18.1% for patients 40 or older, 23.1% for patients over 50, and 25.2% for patients over 60 with a mean of 25.0 months to THA [12].

Age should not be used as an isolated criterium to recommend one or another hip treatment, since significant variability is observed among patients of same age in overall health status, comorbidities, physical activities, requirements, and patient's expectations.

4. Acetabular and femoral abnormalities

Biomechanical abnormalities at the acetabulum and femur are a key factor to consider in borderline cases between hip preservation surgery or THA. Some biomechanical abnormalities contra-indicate or increase the risk of complications for hip arthroscopy and would be better addressed through osteotomy surgeries. However, an osteotomy surgery may not be a good option for a patient when considering the chondral damage, patient age and presence of low back pain. In addition, some patients will not be willing to undergo an osteotomy when considering the surgery magnitude and recovery. Therefore, acetabular and femoral biomechanical abnormalities will influence the decision on conservative management, hip arthroscopy, hip osteotomy or THA. These treatment option should be considered as a continuum of treatment for many patients, as more invasive procedures are recommended when less invasive interventions fail.

4.1 Acetabular dysplasia

The presence of acetabular dysplasia and its severity is to be considered before recommending a hip arthroscopy procedure versus other treatment options. Hip arthroscopy as isolated treatment for moderate to severe acetabular dysplasia has been associated with poor outcomes [14, 15]. However, hip arthroscopy with capsule repair has demonstrated good outcomes for patients with borderline hip dysplasia, traditionally described as lateral center-edge angle between 20° and 25° [16, 17]. Domb et al. reported the results of hip arthroscopy in 22 patients with lateral center-edge angle between 18° and 25°, and no or mild osteoarthritis (Tönnis grade 0 or 1) [16]. The authors utilized a combined imbrication and inferior capsular shift of the iliofemoral ligament to close the hip capsule arthroscopically. Good to excellent results were reported in 77% of the patients at a mean follow-up of 28 months, with 2 patients (9%) requiring revision surgery due to repeat sports injury or trauma [16]. The mean Tönnis angle of 5.8°, within normal limits, and the absence of significant osteoarthritis are important to consider on the results reported by Domb et al. [16]. Fukui et al. described the results of hip arthroscopy in 28 patients with lateral center-edge angle between 15° and 19°, at a mean follow-up of 42 months [17]. Five patients (18%) with a mean joint space <2 mm before hip arthroscopy underwent THA at a mean follow-up of 24 months after the hip arthroscopy [17]. Two patients (7%) required a periacetabular osteotomy to treat dysplasia after failure to improve following hip arthroscopy, while other two patients required a revision hip arthroscopy [17]. The mean Tönnis angle in patients who required periacetabular osteotomy after hip arthroscopy was 21°, while those not requiring PAO had a mean Tönnis angle of 15°. Fukuda et al. concluded that major surgery following hip arthroscopy is more likely for older patients, male, with more severe dysplasia, and with a larger alpha angle and decreased joint space [17]. Uchida et al. studied 28 patients with acetabular dysplasia who underwent hip arthroscopy [18]. The authors reported that patients with a broken Shenton line, femoral neck-shaft angle >140°, lateral center-edge angle <19°, or BMI >23 kg/m2 at the time of surgery are not good candidates for the arthroscopic management of acetabular dysplasia [18]. A major limitation of the studies by Domb, Fukui and Uchida et al. is the lack of consideration for the femoral torsion [16, 17]. Larson et al. reported inferior results of hip arthroscopy in 88 dysplastic hips when compared to non-dysplastic hips treated for femoroacetabular impingement [19]. The authors defined failure as a modified Harris Hip Score (mHHS) ≤70 or eventual pelvic/femoral osteotomy or total hip arthroplasty. At the time of final follow-up, the dysplastic cohort demonstrated a mean mHHS of 81.3 with a mean 15.6-point improvement in mHHS, compared with 88.4 and 24.4 points, respectively, in the femoroacetabular impingement cohort [19]. Larson et al. also reported that increased femoral torsion and psoas tenotomies did not influence the outcomes in hips with acetabular dysplasia [19].

Periacetabular osteotomy (PAO) is another option for patients with acetabular dysplasia that should be considered for some patients to preserve the hip joint, prolong the native hip life, or as a bridge to a THA. Studies on long term results have provided insight on when is too late for a PAO. Matheney et al. reported the outcomes of PAO in 135 hips at an average follow-up of 9 years [20]. Two independent predictors of failure (defined as arthroplasty or a high pain score) were identified: (1) an age of more than thirty-five years and (2) poor or fair preoperative joint congruency [20]. The probability of failure requiring arthroplasty was 14% for hips with no predictors of failure, 36% for those with one predictor (either an age of more than thirty-five years or poor or fair joint congruency), and 95% for those with both predictors [20]. Wells et al. reported the outcomes of PAO in 154 hips at an average of 10.3 years post-operatively [21]. One hundred and twenty-two hips (79%) did not undergo THA and did not have significant hip symptoms at the final follow-up [21]. A higher risk of failure was associated with fair or poor preoperative joint congruency and with overcorrection (a postoperative lateral center-edge angle of >38°) [21].

Association of hip arthroscopy and periacetabular osteotomy is another option of treatment for patients with acetabular dysplasia. Hip arthroscopy after a PAO surgery is required in 3.1–27% according to different authors [22, 23]. In patients with hip dysplasia who fail hip arthroscopy, PAO has been shown to be successful and results did not differ from patients who undergo PAO as index procedure [24].

A frequent question from patients is if undergoing a PAO or hip arthroscopy would decrease the chances of success for a THA procedure in the future. Considering THA after a PAO, the medical literature is controversial. Amanatullah et al. reported no difference in complication, revision rates or clinical results for THA in dysplastic patients with or without prior PAO [25]. Osawa et al. reported poorer clinical outcomes of THA in patients with prior PAO compared to dysplastic patients without PAO, although there was no difference in revision or complication between the groups [26]. Both studies observed increased rates of acetabular component malposition in hips with prior PAO [25, 26]. In regards to results of THA following hip arthroscopy, Lemme et al. reported that patients who underwent THA more than 1 year after hip arthroscopy were at no increased risk for surgical or medical complications [27]. However, increased risk of dislocation (OR 1.75; CI 1.05–2.87; P = .03) and aseptic loosening (OR 2.18; CI 1.06–4.49; P = .03) was observed if the THA was performed <1 year after the hip arthroscopy [27]. THA <1 year after hip arthroscopy was also associated with increased risk for needing revision THA at 2 years (OR 1.92; CI 1.07–3.36; P = .02) and 4 years (OR 2.05; CI 1.17–3.53; P = .01) after THA.

The severity of hip dysplasia is usually defined by the morphologic features of the acetabular roof. However, abnormalities of the acetabular horns and sagittal orientation of the acetabulum are also frequent and have not been studied regarding the results of hip preservation surgery. Further studies are necessary to define if hips with antero-inferior or posteroinferior acetabular undercoverage have inferior results with hip arthroscopic procedures (**Figure 3**). Abnormal acetabular slope (sagittal orientation of the acetabulum) is another factor that requires further investigation when recommending a preservation or reconstruction procedure (**Figure 4**).

4.2 Femoral torsion and acetabular version abnormalities

Assessment in three planes is a basic requirement for any project in engineering. The hip joint is a complex biomechanical construct, and evaluation in three anatomical planes should be completed before any surgical recommendation. The imaging assessment of the hip joint has historically neglected the axial plane due to the inherent limitations of radiographs. Currently, the broad availability of MRI and CT to orthopedic surgeons makes it difficult to justify the lack of imaging assessment in three anatomical planes (axial, coronal and sagittal). The femoral torsion is one of the hip parameters assessed in the axial plane and has not received the necessary attention by clinicians and researchers in the orthopedic field. Increased femoral torsion is associated with decreased extension and external rotation, and increased internal rotation of the hip [30–35]. Decreased femoral torsion is associated with increased external rotation and decreased internal rotation of the hip [30–33]. Effects of abnormal femoral torsion on the lumbopelvic biomechanics have also been reported, and can be estimated by the hip-spine extension and flexion tests on physical examination [36, 37].

A recent systematic review on the effect of acetabular version on outcomes of hip arthroscopy concluded that surgery in patients with acetabular retroversion resulted in no difference in functional outcomes compared with patients with normal acetabular version [38]. The medical literature has controversial results on the influence of

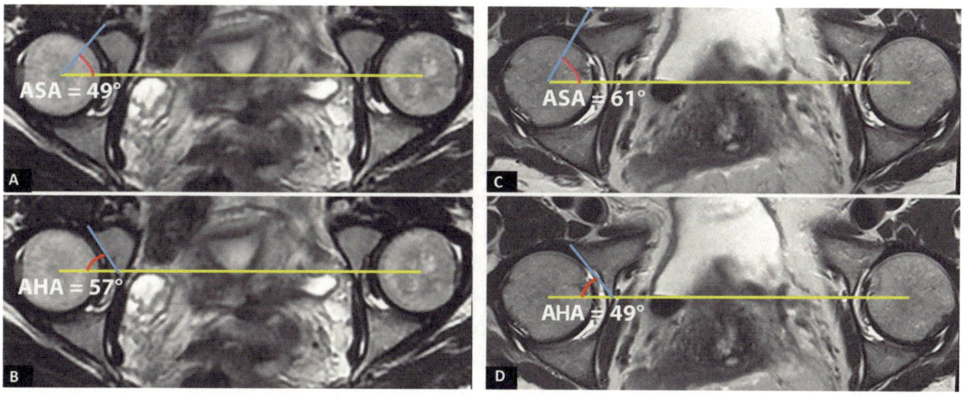

Figure 3.
Antero-inferior hip instability. A and B) right hip with anteroinferior instability observed arthroscopically, with decreased anterior sector angle (ASA < 58°) and increased anterior horn angle (AHA > 50°); C and D) right hip with normal anterior acetabular horn morphology, with normal ASA and normal AHA. Reprinted from Hatem et al. Anteroinferior hip instability in flexion during dynamic arthroscopic examination is associated with abnormal anterior acetabular horn [28].

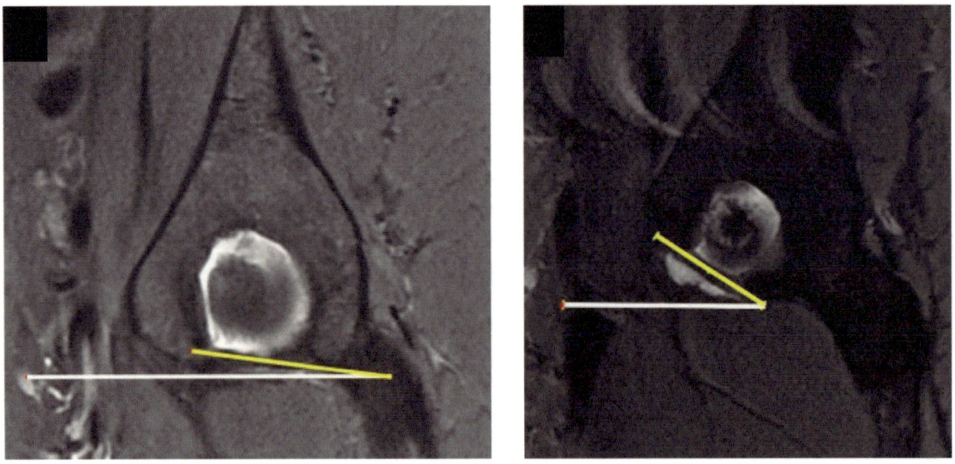

(A) (B)

Figure 4.
Sagittal slice of a hip magnetic resonance arthrogram demonstrating the acetabular slope. (A) Hip with decreased acetabular slope (8°); B) hip with increased acetabular slope (33°). Reprinted from Hatem et al. spinopelvic parameters do not predict the sagittal orientation of the acetabulum [29].

femoral torsion on hip arthroscopy results. Fabricant et al. observed less improvement following hip arthroscopy in patients with <5° of femoral torsion compared with patients with normal and increased femoral torsion [39]. In contrast, two studies did not report decreased femoral torsion to be a negative prognostic factor for hip arthroscopy [40, 41]. Both studies did not include functional assessment of lumbar spine. Chaharbakhshi et al. reported that patients with combined borderline dysplasia and femoral torsion ≥20° demonstrated significant improvements after hip arthroscopy, despite the inferior results when compared with a control group with normal version and acetabular coverage [42]. Jackson et al. found that femoral torsion >18° was not a negative prognostic factor for hip arthroscopy [43]. Fabricant et al. described inferior results (modified Harris Hip Score) of hip arthroscopy with psoas tenotomy for patients with >25° of femoral torsion [44]. Part of the controversy on the results is explained by differences on how to measure femoral torsion among the studies and the definition of normal, increased or decreased femoral torsion. Most studies on the effect of femoral torsion on hip arthroscopy consider decreased femoral torsion as <5° and increased femoral torsion as >20° [38]. The method utilized for the measurement of the femoral torsion is to be considered for the purpose of comparison to other studies [45–47]. Increasing values for femoral torsion are observed by measuring the femoral neck orientation more distally, and differences of 10° or more among the methods are particularly frequent in patients with excessive femoral torsion [46]. Until the controversy is resolved, it is recommendable to assess femoral torsion and acetabular version for McKibbin's index as routine for patients with hip symptoms.

Femoral derotation osteotomy is to be considered for patients with abnormal femoral torsion, particularly those with failed hip arthroscopy and with low back pain. Tönnis and Heinecke reported satisfactory results of PFDO in 17 patients with decreased femoral torsion and painful hip joints [31]. Another study showing improvement in hip function with PFDO was published by Buly et al., who reported a mean improvement of 27 points in the mHHS following 55 derotation osteotomies in 43 patients [48]. Hatem et al. reported 34 patients who underwent proximal femoral derotation osteotomy [37]. Improvement in the mHHS above the minimum clinically important difference (MCID) was observed in 33 hips (89%). In a subgroup of 14 consecutive patients assessed with Oswestry disability index (ODI), the ODI improved from a mean of 45% before the PFDO to 22% at final follow-up [37].

The orthopedic surgeon might consider that extreme values of femoral torsion will have higher biomechanical effects. Therefore, the influence of femoral torsion >30° or below 0° is more clinically significant than the normal range values presented in medical literature. Ligamentous structures play a role on the biomechanical effects of increased and decreased femoral torsion and further studies are needed to better understand the relationship between the iliofemoral ligament and femoral torsion. The patient body habitus and frame will have an influence on strain tolerance to abnormal femoral torsion. Physical examination is essential to determine the biomechanical effects of abnormal femoral torsion and to guide treatment, particularly testing gait in different hip rotation and the hip spine-extension test (**Figure 5**) [49]. The femoral torsion should be considered factor when deciding between hip preservation surgery and THA. In older patients, abnormal femoral torsion may add up to other negative prognostic factors towards a recommendation for THA.

4.3 Ischiofemoral impingement

Ischiofemoral impingement is associated with limitation in hip extension. A more aggressive treatment approach may be recommended for individuals with secondary biomechanical effects of ischiofemoral impingement as low back and pelvic pain. Gómez-Hoyos et al. simulated a hip extension deficit with an ischiofemoral impingement model to evaluate a primary hip-spine effect due to the limited terminal hip extension produced by the hip pathology [50]. Resultant data described significant increase in lumbar facet joint loading during the impingement state, as compared to the native state for L3-L4 and L4-L5 spine segments. An average 30% increase in facet joint overload was observed between impinged state and native state [50].

Conservative treatment for ischiofemoral impingement includes avoidance of impingement positions, correction of leg length inequality, abductor strengthening, correction of foot hyperpronation and guided injections. Surgical treatment options are indicated when conservative treatment is insufficient: endoscopic lesser trochanter plasty and resection; open lesser trochanter resection; ischioplasty; distal transfer of the lesser trochanter; proximal femoral osteotomy -varus and derotation osteotomy; and finally total hip arthroplasty. The orthopedic surgeon should consider the presence of ischiofemoral impingement in borderline cases between hip preservation surgery and THA. Individuals with ischiofemoral impingement and associated advanced chondral damage of the hip joint are better suited for THA. Total hip arthroplasty is also an alternative to address ischiofemoral impingement in hips with mechanical failure from multiple biomechanical abnormalities, including hip dysplasia and abnormal femoral torsion. A posterior approach allows the repair of hamstring avulsion at the ischial tuberosity, often observed as a result from the ischiofemoral impingement. The presence of contra-lateral hip disease, knee osteoarthritis, and lumbar spine abnormalities reinforce the indication of total hip arthroplasty to treat ischiofemoral impingement. The orthopedic surgeon performing a hip joint replacement in individuals with IFI must be aware of all parameters in the coronal, axial and sagittal planes for the correction of all biomechanical abnormalities. Testing hip extension intra-operatively is fundamental in patients with IFI undergoing total hip arthroplasty through either anterior, lateral or posterior approach.

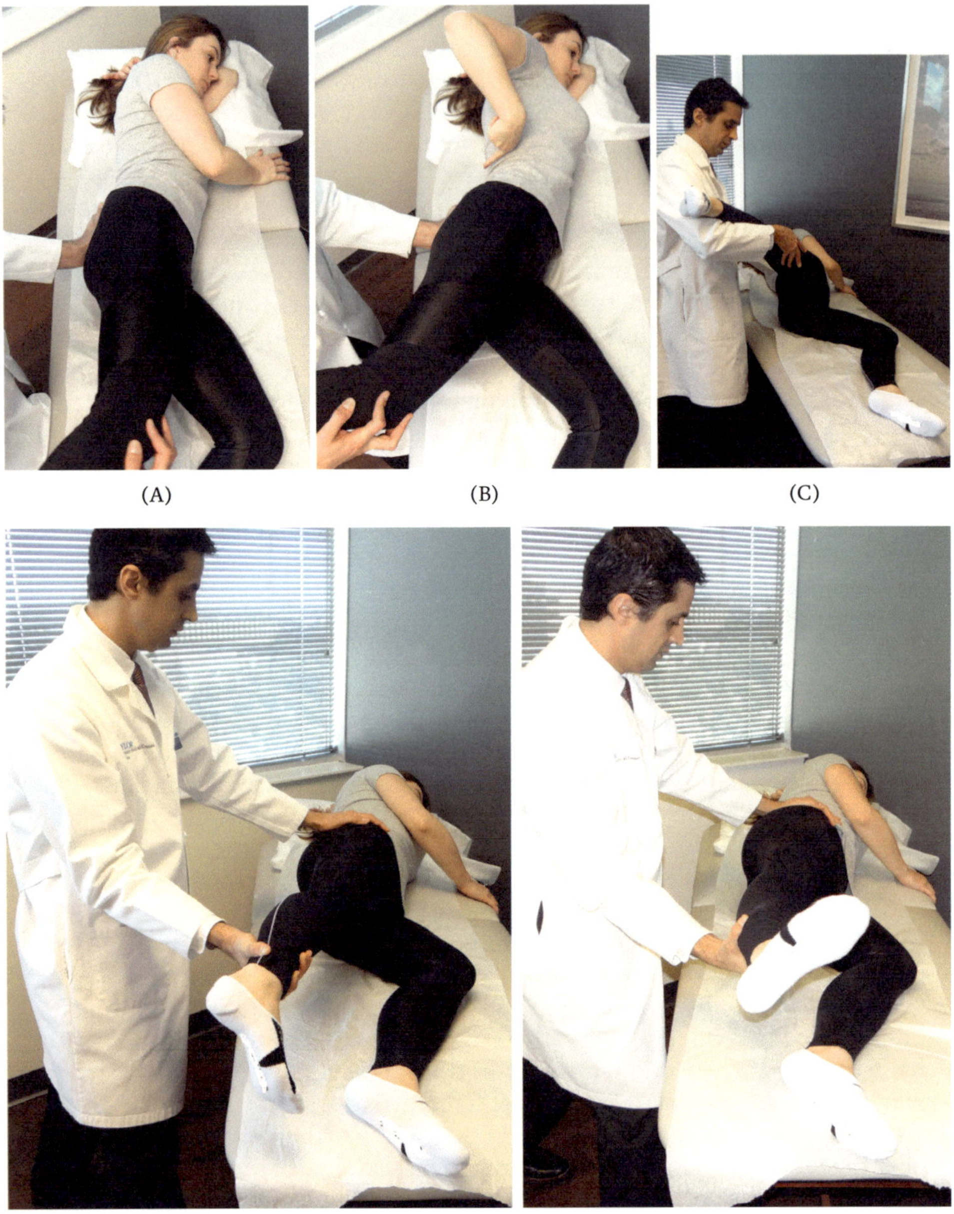

(A) (B) (C)

(D) (E)

Figure 5.
Hip-spine extension test. (A) the examined hip is brought into terminal hip extension in neutral abduction and rotation while the examiner observes the pelvis and lumbar spine; (B) a positive result is the recreation of low back pain with associated pelvic and lumbar movement in adaptation to the limited hip extension; (C) adding abduction to extension allows the hip to extend without secondary effects at the pelvis and lumbar spine in patients with ischiofemoral impingement; (D) adding internal rotation gives clearance for the extension of the hip in cases of increased femoral anteversion. Conversely, due to premature coupling, internal rotation increases the lumbar and pelvic accommodation in hips with decreased femoral version or retroversion; (E) adding external rotation gives clearance for the extension of the hip in cases of decreased femoral anteversion or retroversion. Conversely, due to premature coupling, external rotation increases the lumbar and pelvic accommodation in hips with increased femoral anteversion.

5. Presence of low back pain

Hip reconstruction surgery has the potential to restore hip mobility to normal levels and remove the secondary effects of limited hip motion on the lumbar spine. Improvement in low back pain after THA has been consistently reported. Parvizi et al. studied 170 patients with low back pain prior to undergoing THA [51]. Postoperatively, 66% (113) patients reported complete resolution of low back pain [51]. Of the 57 patients whose back pain did not resolve postoperatively, 38 had prior suspected or diagnosed spine disorders [51]. Chimenti et al. reported that 60.5% of patients who underwent THA had at least mild back pain preoperatively, and 58.4% of these patients experienced improvement in low back pain of at least 1 degree difference (e.g. moderate to mild) [52]. Notably, 80% of patients who indicated severe low back pain preoperatively showed some degree of pain improvement after THA [52]. Okuzu et al. reported that low back pain improved in 62.9% of patients after THA [53]. Persistent low back pain in the remaining 37.1% of patients after THA was shown to be associated with biomechanical abnormalities of the spine, such as sagittal spinal imbalance and high Cobb angle [53]. A study by Ran et al. examined changes in low back pain after THA in patients with lumbar degenerative disease, and observed a decreased on VAS for pain from 4.13 ± 1.37 preoperatively to 1.90 ± 1.44 postoperatively [54].

Patients with existing spinal pathologies present higher rates of complications after THA. Blizzard et al. conducted a review of the Medicare Standard Analytical Files from 2005 to 2012 [55]. The authors reported that patients with lumbosacral spondylosis, lumbar disc herniation, lumbar degenerative disc disease, and spondylolisthesis prior to THA had increased risk of post-operative complications such as prosthetic joint dislocation, periprosthetic fractures, periprosthetic infections, early revision THA, and wound complications [55].

Less evidence is available on hip preservation surgery and low back pain. Beck et al. reported that patients with a history of lumbosacral pathology (i.e. stenosis, fracture, prior surgery, and disc pathology) had significantly lower Hip Outcome Scores (activities of daily living subscale and sports subscale), modified Harris Hip Score, and visual analog scale pain two years after hip arthroscopy [56]. In contrast, in a cohort of 48 elite athletes with low back pain who underwent hip arthroscopy, Jiminez et al. reported that 79% did not report low back pain postoperatively at a mean follow-up of 53 months [57]. Endoscopic treatment for ischiofemoral impingement has also been associated with improvement in low back pain. Hatem et al. studied 31 patients with ischiofemoral impingement and low back pain who were treated with endoscopic partial lesser trochanter resection [58]. The authors reported a decrease in low back pain above the minimal clinically important difference in 2 of 3 patients after partial resection of the lesser trochanter [58]. Surgical correction of abnormal femoral torsion with derotation osteotomy has also been associated with improvement in low back pain. Hatem et al. reported that 14 patients with abnormal femoral torsion and LBP who underwent femoral derotation osteotomy demonstrated improved Oswestry disability index scores from 45% ± 16% (mean ± SD) before the PFDO to 22% ± 17% (mean ± SD) at mean follow-up of 24 months [37]. Nine (64.3%) of the 14 patients presented improvement in the Oswestry disability index above the minimal clinically important difference [37].

6. Other factors

The decision between hip preservation surgery and THA for borderline cases is also influenced by the following factors barely addressed in medical literature: patient expectations, abnormalities in additional hip layers, contra-lateral hip disease, profession and physical activities, commitment to rehabilitation, family support, chronicity of pain, opioid use, comorbidities, and physician-related aspects. Despite the lack of scientific evidence on those factors, the authors of the current chapter decided to share their impressions after combined decades of experience on deciding if conservative treatment, hip preservation surgery, or THA would be the most appropriate.

The concept of hip layers is very useful for the orthopedic surgeon to identify and organize diagnosis in patients with hip abnormalities, and to relate those to the patient expectations. The hip abnormalities can be categorized in the following layers: osteochondral, capsulolabral, musculotendinous, neurovascular, and kinematic chain. The fifth layer represents the link between the hip, pelvis, lumbar spine, CORE and distal lower extremity. Most patients with hip symptoms will have problems in more than one layer, which can be related or unrelated. For example, patients with acetabular dysplasia often have associated gluteus medius and minimus tendinitis as result of excess work required from the abductors. The correction of the osseous abnormalities may or not result in improvement of the conditions in other layers. Each diagnosis and potential improvement or not with surgery must be shared with patients, so they can understand the decision process and be aware that some problems/symptoms may not get better with surgery. Most patients believe their hip problem can be cured and expect to be asymptomatic at the end of treatment. This outcome is unlikely for hip pathologies and patients will have a more realistic expectation if they are instructed before surgery about a multilayer diagnosis.

The hip joint is the center of human body movement, and functional hips are required for most activities of daily living. When both hips become symptomatic, life can become particularly challenging. In most hip preservation surgeries, the operated hip will require at least 3 to 6 months of protected activities, and the non-operated hip may become more symptomatic. A THA is usually more foreseeable under the rehabilitation point of view and is a better option for most patients with bilateral hip symptoms and borderline case between preservation and THA. Patient profession is another important factor in borderline cases. Consider the following clinical scenario: a 50-year-old male farmer with symptomatic labral tear and grade 1–2 osteoarthritis with Harris hip score of 60 and Oswestry score of 20%, associated contra-lateral hip and low back pain, need to return to work in weeks after surgery, and average of 2 miles walked daily. Even if imaging studies do not contra-indicate hip preservation surgery, this patient's profession and clinical scenario indicate that a THA might be a treatment option for him. Conservative treatment or hip arthroscopy could be a more appropriate option to an office worker with the same clinical scenario except for the profession. Per our experience, non-athlete patients with higher physical demands on their job tend to be less satisfied with hip arthroscopy and preservation surgeries. Not only the profession and work are to be considered, but also the physical requirements of leisure and family requirements. Commitment to rehabilitation and family support are factors often overlooked by patients and physicians before making a treatment decision for hip pathologies. Because of the demands involved with recovery processes after hip surgery, the patient may be limited for regular home tasks and requires the support of family. Socioeconomic factors are important to consider when deciding between hip preservation surgery or THA. Hip preservation surgery requires months and sometimes years to reach the maximum improvement, particularly in patients with multilayer hip problems.

The chronicity of hip pain experienced prior can play a role in deciding which treatment route to pursue. Garbuz et al. found that patients who waited more than 6 months before THA had a 50% decrease in the odds of achieving a better-than-expected outcome as measured by the Western Ontario McMaster Universities Osteoarthritis Index (WOMAC) when compared to patients with 0–6 months delay [59]. Moreover, each additional month delay after 6 months was associated with 8% additional decrease in odds of achieving a better-than-expected WOMAC score [59]. Similar decreases in clinical outcome scores have been shown with increased preoperative duration of pain in arthroscopic patients. Kunze et al. reported that hip pain from femoroacetabular impingement for 12–24 months in duration preceding surgery was associated with worse postoperative outcomes compared to hip pain with a duration of 3–6 months before surgery [60]. Basques et al. reported similar results: patients with femoroacetabular impingement and more than 2 years of preoperative hip pain have significantly higher 2-year VAS-pain scores, along with significantly lower HOS-ADL, HOS-SS, and mHHS scores after hip arthroscopy [61].

Preoperative opioid use has been associated with less favorable postoperative outcomes after hip preservation surgery and THA. Weick et al. reported that THA patients with >60 days of preoperative opioid use, compared to opioid-naïve patients and patients with <60 days preoperative use, had increased odds of readmission at 30 days postoperatively (OR = 1.46, CI: 1.36–1.57) and needing revision surgery at 1 year (OR = 2.19, CI: 1.84–2.62) [62]. The odds of requiring revision surgery was found to be even greater by the 3-year mark (OR = 1.90, CI: 1.64–2.20) [62]. Zusmanovich et al. reported that patients who regularly used opioids for isolated hip pain within 6 months before hip arthroscopy had higher 1-year postoperative VAS scores compared to opioid-naïve patients (6.1 ± 3.1 vs. 1.5 ± 1.6, respectively) ($p < .001$) [63]. At 2-year postoperatively, mHHS was significantly lower in the study cohort of opioid users compared to opioid-naïve group (55.4 ± 19.6 vs. 80.4 ± 12.8, respectively) ($p < .001$) [63]. Nazzal et al. reported that 2501 hip arthroscopy patients who preoperatively were taking >5 oral morphine equivalents had statistically significantly increased odds of prolonged opioid use (i.e. ≥2 opioid prescriptions) in the 6- to 12-month postoperative period (OR, 10.45; $p < 0.001$) compared to 19,633 patients who took fewer oral morphine equivalents [64]. These patients were also shown to have increased odds of 3-year revision surgery (both hip arthroscopy and total hip arthroplasty: OR = 2.14, $p < 0.001$ and OR = 2.04, $p = 0.001$, respectively) [64]. The reversibility of the negative effects of opioid use in hip surgery results has not been defined yet, i.e., does a patient on chronic opioid use benefit from stopping it before a hip surgery? Until further evidence is available, patients might be instructed to work on strategies along with their pain management providers aiming to decrease or stop opioid use before elective hip surgery.

The presence of additional medical conditions may influence the outcome and success of hip reconstruction and preservation procedures. Loth et al. reported that THA patients with ≥1 comorbidity on the Charlson comorbidity index (CCI), pain from other joints, or BMI > 30 kg/m2 did not have significantly different postoperative improvements in pain and joint function when compared to THA patients with no comorbidities [65]. However, patients with comorbidities were still found to have lower general health scores (mean of 39.1 vs. 44.9) as measured by the Short Form-12 (SF-12) ($p < .001$) [65]. Mannion et al. reported that greater comorbidity was associated with increased odds of a complication and (independently) slightly worse patient-rated outcome 12 months after THA [66]. Fewer studies have investigated the relationship between comorbidities and hip arthroscopy outcomes. Perets et al. reported diabetes mellitus is not significantly associated with worse outcomes in hip arthroscopy cases for treatment of femoroacetabular impingement and labral tears [67]. The psychological status and psychiatric conditions are also to be considered in patients with chronic hip pain. Patients often enter in a pain cycle bolstering the effects of hip pain and limitation in their lives. Sochacki et al. reported that patients with minimal or mild depressive symptoms have better preoperative and postoperative outcomes and are more likely to obtain substantial clinical benefit from surgery than patients with moderate to severe depressive symptoms [68]. Martin et al. reported a high prevalence of patients with symptoms of depression (28%) and severe depression (11%) among 781 patients who underwent hip arthroscopy [69]. The high prevalence of depression in patients with chronic hip pain reinforces the importance of optimal hip function for a healthy mental status. Buller et al. reported the existing diagnosis of depression, dementia, or schizophrenia in THA patients is significantly associated with increased odds of adverse effects after THA (i.e. wound complication, shock, acute renal failure, etc.) [70]. Consultation with a pain psychologist is helpful for patients with chronic hip pain to address the mind effects of chronic pain, and to identify patients whose psychological status may impede improvement after hip surgery.

7. Summary

Evaluation of the anatomy and biomechanics through clinical, functional, and triplanar imaging assessments is essential on decision-making for conservative treatment, hip preservation surgery and THA. The concept of hip layers is very useful for the orthopedic surgeon to identify and organize diagnosis and treatment plan in patients with hip abnormalities, and to relate those to the patient expectations. The effects of abnormal hip biomechanics on the spine-pelvis-CORE need to be considered when treating hip conditions. Hip diseases are treated and rarely cured. The treatment of hip diseases should be approached in a stepwise fashion, starting with education, accommodation, medication, physical therapy, mental rehabilitation, and injections. When conservative measures fail, the surgical treatment decision will be influenced by a comprehensive history and physical examination with triplanar imaging osseous assessment with discussion of patient expectations and commitment. In the future, the influence of hip treatment on hip-spine-pelvic-CORE will play a greater role on decision-making process.

Author details

Munif Hatem[1*], Richard Feng[2], Srino Bharam[3] and Hal David Martin[4]

1 Hip Preservation Center - Baylor Scott and White Research Institute, Dallas, United States

2 Texas A&M College of Medicine, Dallas, United States

3 New York Hip Preservation and Groin Center at Lenox Hill Hospital of Northwell Health, New York, United States

4 Hip Preservation Center at Baylor University Medical Center at Dallas, Dallas, United States

*Address all correspondence to: munifhatem@gmail.com

References

[1] Kemp JL, MacDonald D, Collins NJ, Hatton AL, Crossley KM. Hip arthroscopy in the setting of hip osteoarthritis: Systematic review of outcomes and progression to hip arthroplasty. Clinical Orthopaedics. 2015;**473**(3):1055-1073

[2] McCarthy JC, Jarrett BT, Ojeifo O, Lee JA, Bragdon CR. What factors influence long-term survivorship after hip arthroscopy? Clinical Orthopaedics. 2011;**469**(2):362-371

[3] Horisberger M, Brunner A, Herzog RF. Arthroscopic treatment of femoral acetabular impingement in patients with preoperative generalized degenerative changes. Arthroscopy: The Journal of Arthroscopic & Related Official Publication of the Arthroscopy Association North America and the International Arthroscopy Association. 2010;**26**(5):623-629

[4] Zimmerer A, Ramoser A, Streit M, Janz V, Sobau C, Wassilew GI, et al. Osteoarthrosis, advanced age, and female sex are risk factors for inferior outcomes after hip arthroscopy and labral debridement for Femoroacetabular impingement syndrome: Case series with minimum 10-year follow-up. Arthroscopy. 2021;**37**(6):1822-1828.e1

[5] Bessa FS, Williams BT, Polce EM, Maheshwer B, Williams JC, Nho SJ, et al. No differences in hip joint space measurements between Weightbearing or supine anteroposterior pelvic radiographs. Arthroscopy: The Journal of Arthroscopic & Related Official Publication of the Arthroscopy Association North America and the International Arthroscopy Association. 2020;**36**(11):2843-2848

[6] Philippon MJ, Briggs KK, Yen Y-M, Kuppersmith DA. Outcomes following hip arthroscopy for femoroacetabular impingement with associated chondrolabral dysfunction: Minimum two-year follow-up. Journal of Bone and Joint Surgery. British Volume (London). 2009;**91**(1):16-23

[7] Rosinsky PJ, Chen JW, Lall AC, Wojnowski NM, Shapira J, Maldonado DR, et al. Can radiographic joint space accurately predict chondral damage during hip arthroscopy? A cross-sectional analysis. Arthroscopy: The Journal of Arthroscopic & Related Official Publication of the Arthroscopy Association North America and the International Arthroscopy Association. 2020;**36**(6):1565-1572.e1

[8] Peters CL, Schabel K, Anderson L, Erickson J. Open treatment of femoroacetabular impingement is associated with clinical improvement and low complication rate at short-term followup. Clinical Orthopaedics. 2010;**468**(2):504-510

[9] Eijer H, Hogervorst T. Femoroacetabular impingement causes osteoarthritis of the hip by migration and micro-instability of the femoral head. Medical Hypotheses. 2017;**104**:93-96

[10] Malik AT, Jain N, Scharschmidt TJ, Glassman AH, Khan SN. Primary hip arthroscopy and conversion to total hip arthroplasty: Trends and survival analysis in the Medicare population. Hip International Journal of Clinical Experience Research Hip Pathology Therapy. 2020;**31**:1120700020951171

[11] Martin SD, Abraham PF, Varady NH, Nazal MR, Conaway W, Quinlan NJ, et al. Hip arthroscopy versus physical therapy

for the treatment of symptomatic acetabular labral tears in patients older than 40 years: A randomized controlled trial. The American Journal of Sports Medicine. 2021;**49**(5):1199-1208

[12] Horner NS, Ekhtiari S, Simunovic N, Safran MR, Philippon MJ, Ayeni OR. Hip arthroscopy in patients age 40 or older: A systematic review. Arthroscopy: The Journal of Arthroscopic & Related Official Publication of the Arthroscopy Association North America and the International Arthroscopy Association. 2017;**33**(2):464-475.e3

[13] Sharfman ZT, Safran N, Amar E, Varshneya K, Safran MR, Rath E. Age-adjusted normative values for hip patient-reported outcome measures. The American Journal of Sports Medicine. 2022;**50**(1):79-84

[14] Ross JR, Clohisy JC, Baca G, Sink E, Investigators ANCHOR. Patient and disease characteristics associated with hip arthroscopy failure in acetabular dysplasia. The Journal of Arthroplasty. 2014;**29**(9 Suppl):160-163

[15] Adler KL, Giordano BD. The utility of hip arthroscopy in the setting of acetabular dysplasia: A systematic review. Arthroscopy: The Journal of Arthroscopic & Related Official Publication of the Arthroscopy Association North America and the International Arthroscopy Association. 2019;**35**(1):237-248

[16] Domb BG, Stake CE, Lindner D, El-Bitar Y, Jackson TJ. Arthroscopic capsular plication and labral preservation in borderline hip dysplasia: Two-year clinical outcomes of a surgical approach to a challenging problem. The American Journal of Sports Medicine. 2013;**41**(11):2591-2598

[17] Fukui K, Trindade CA, Briggs KK, Philippon MJ. Arthroscopy of the hip for patients with mild to moderate developmental dysplasia of the hip and femoroacetabular impingement: Outcomes following hip arthroscopy for treatment of chondrolabral damage. The Bone & Joint Journal. 2015 Oct;**97-B**(10):1316-1321

[18] Uchida S, Utsunomiya H, Mori T, Taketa T, Nishikino S, Nakamura T, et al. Clinical and radiographic predictors for worsened clinical outcomes after hip arthroscopic labral preservation and capsular closure in developmental dysplasia of the hip. The American Journal of Sports Medicine. 2016;**44**(1):28-38

[19] Larson CM, Ross JR, Stone RM, Samuelson KM, Schelling EF, Giveans MR, et al. Arthroscopic Management of Dysplastic hip Deformities: Predictors of success and failures with comparison to an arthroscopic FAI cohort. The American Journal of Sports Medicine. 2016;**44**(2):447-453

[20] Matheney T, Kim Y-J, Zurakowski D, Matero C, Millis M. Intermediate to long-term results following the Bernese periacetabular osteotomy and predictors of clinical outcome. The Journal of Bone and Joint Surgery. American Volume. 2009;**91**(9):2113-2123

[21] Wells J, Schoenecker P, Duncan S, Goss CW, Thomason K, Clohisy JC. Intermediate-term hip survivorship and patient-reported outcomes of Periacetabular osteotomy: The Washington university experience. The Journal of Bone and Joint Surgery. American Volume. 2018;**100**(3):218-225

[22] Hartig-Andreasen C, Troelsen A, Thillemann TM, Gelineck J, Søballe K. Risk factors for the need of hip arthroscopy following periacetabular osteotomy. Journal of Hip Preservation Surgery. 2015;**2**(4):374-384

[23] Cvetanovich GL, Heyworth BE, Murray K, Yen Y-M, Kocher MS, Millis MB. Hip arthroscopy in patients with recurrent pain following Bernese periacetabular osteotomy for acetabular dysplasia: Operative findings and clinical outcomes. Journal of Hip Preservation Surgery. 2015;**2**(3):295-302

[24] Kain MSH, Novais EN, Vallim C, Millis MB, Kim Y-J. Periacetabular osteotomy after failed hip arthroscopy for labral tears in patients with acetabular dysplasia. The Journal of Bone and Joint Surgery. American Volume. 2011;**93**(Suppl 2):57-61

[25] Amanatullah DF, Stryker L, Schoenecker P, Taunton MJ, Clohisy JC, Trousdale RT, et al. Similar clinical outcomes for THAs with and without prior periacetabular osteotomy. Clinical Orthopaedics. 2015;**473**(2):685-691

[26] Osawa Y, Hasegawa Y, Seki T, Amano T, Higuchi Y, Ishiguro N. Significantly poor outcomes of Total hip arthroplasty after failed Periacetabular osteotomy. The Journal of Arthroplasty. 2016;**31**(9):1904-1909

[27] Lemme NJ, Veeramani A, Yang DS, Tabaddor RR, Daniels AH, Cohen EM. Total hip arthroplasty after hip arthroscopy has increased complications and revision risk. The Journal of Arthroplasty. 2021;**36**(12):3922-3927.e2

[28] Hatem MA, Helal A, Khoury AN, Martin HD. Anteroinferior hip instability in flexion during dynamic arthroscopic examination is associated with abnormal anterior acetabular horn. Orthopaedic Journal of Sports Medicine. 2020;**8**(12):2325967120965564

[29] Hatem M, Nimmons SJ, Khoury AN, Martin HD. Spinopelvic parameters do not predict the sagittal orientation of the acetabulum. Orthopaedic Journal of Sports Medicine. 2020;**8**(10):2325967120957420

[30] Tönnis D, Heinecke A. Acetabular and femoral anteversion: Relationship with osteoarthritis of the hip. The Journal of Bone and Joint Surgery. American Volume. 1999;**81**(12):1747-1770

[31] Tönnis D, Heinecke A. Diminished femoral antetorsion syndrome: A cause of pain and osteoarthritis. Journal of Pediatric Orthopedics. 1991;**11**(4):419-431

[32] Kraeutler MJ, Chadayammuri V, Garabekyan T, Mei-Dan O. Femoral version abnormalities significantly outweigh effect of cam impingement on hip internal rotation. The Journal of Bone and Joint Surgery. American Volume. 2018;**100**(3):205-210

[33] Chadayammuri V, Garabekyan T, Bedi A, Pascual-Garrido C, Rhodes J, O'Hara J, et al. Passive hip range of motion predicts femoral torsion and acetabular version. The Journal of Bone and Joint Surgery. American Volume. 2016;**98**(2):127-134

[34] Siebenrock KA, Steppacher SD, Haefeli PC, Schwab JM, Tannast M. Valgus hip with high antetorsion causes pain through posterior extraarticular FAI. Clinical Orthopaedics. 2013;**471**(12):3774-3780

[35] Morris WZ, Fowers CA, Weinberg DS, Millis MB, Tu L-A, Liu RW. Hip morphology predicts posterior hip impingement in a cadaveric model. Hip International Journal of Clinical Experience Research Hip Pathology Therapy. 2019;**29**(3):322-327

[36] Khoury AN, Hatem M, Bowler J, Martin HD. Hip-spine syndrome: Rationale for ischiofemoral

impingement, femoroacetabular impingement and abnormal femoral torsion leading to low back pain. Journal of Hip Preservation Surgery. 2020;7(3):390-400

[37] Hatem M, Khoury AN, Erickson LR, Jones AL, Martin HD. Femoral Derotation osteotomy improves hip and spine function in patients with increased or decreased femoral torsion. Arthroscopy: The Journal of Arthroscopic & Related Official Publication of the Arthroscopy Association North America and the International Arthroscopy Association. 2021;**37**(1):111-123

[38] Wang CK, Cohen D, Kay J, Almasri M, Simunovic N, Cardenas-Nylander C, et al. The effect of femoral and acetabular version on outcomes following hip arthroscopy: A systematic review. The Journal of Bone and Joint Surgery. American Volume. 2022;**104**(3):271-283

[39] Fabricant PD, Fields KG, Taylor SA, Magennis E, Bedi A, Kelly BT. The effect of femoral and acetabular version on clinical outcomes after arthroscopic femoroacetabular impingement surgery. The Journal of Bone and Joint Surgery. American Volume. 2015;**97**(7):537-543

[40] Lall AC, Battaglia MR, Maldonado DR, Perets I, Laseter JR, Go CC, et al. Does femoral retroversion adversely affect outcomes after hip arthroscopy for Femoroacetabular impingement syndrome? A midterm analysis. Arthroscopy: The Journal of Arthroscopic & Related Official Publication of the Arthroscopy Association North America and the International Arthroscopy Association. 2019;**35**(11):3035-3046

[41] Ferro FP, Ho CP, Briggs KK, Philippon MJ. Patient-centered outcomes after hip arthroscopy for femoroacetabular impingement and labral tears are not different in patients with normal, high, or low femoral version. Arthroscopy: The Journal of Arthroscopic & Related Official Publication of the Arthroscopy Association North America and the International Arthroscopy Association. 2015;**31**(3):454-459

[42] Chaharbakhshi EO, Hartigan DE, Perets I, Domb BG. Is hip arthroscopy effective in patients with combined excessive femoral Anteversion and borderline dysplasia? A match-controlled study. The American Journal of Sports Medicine. 2019;**47**(1):123-130

[43] Jackson TJ, Lindner D, El-Bitar YF, Domb BG. Effect of femoral anteversion on clinical outcomes after hip arthroscopy. Arthroscopy: The Journal of Arthroscopic & Related Official Publication of the Arthroscopy Association North America and the International Arthroscopy Association. 2015;**31**(1):35-41

[44] Fabricant PD, Bedi A, De La Torre K, Kelly BT. Clinical outcomes after arthroscopic psoas lengthening: The effect of femoral version. Arthroscopy: The Journal of Arthroscopic & Related Official Publication of the Arthroscopy Association North America and the International Arthroscopy Association. 2012;**28**(7):965-971

[45] Kaiser P, Attal R, Kammerer M, Thauerer M, Hamberger L, Mayr R, et al. Significant differences in femoral torsion values depending on the CT measurement technique. Archives of Orthopaedic and Trauma Surgery. 2016;**136**(9):1259-1264

[46] Schmaranzer F, Lerch TD, Siebenrock KA, Tannast M, Steppacher SD. Differences in femoral torsion among various measurement

methods increase in hips with excessive femoral torsion. Clinical Orthopaedics. 2019;**477**(5):1073-1083

[47] Sugano N, Noble PC, Kamaric E. A comparison of alternative methods of measuring femoral anteversion. Journal of Computer Assisted Tomography. 1998;**22**(4):610-614

[48] Buly RL, Sosa BR, Poultsides LA, Caldwell E, Rozbruch SR. Femoral Derotation osteotomy in adults for version abnormalities. The Journal of the American Academy of Orthopaedic Surgeons. 2018;**26**(19):e416-e425

[49] Hatem M, Khoury A, Martin HD. Physical examination of the hip and pelvis. In: Hip Arthroscopy and Hip Joint Preservation Surgery. 2nd ed. Gewerbestrasse, Switzerland: Springer; 2022

[50] Gómez-Hoyos J, Khoury A, Schröder R, Johnson E, Palmer IJ, Martin HD. The hip-spine effect: A biomechanical study of Ischiofemoral impingement effect on lumbar facet joints. Arthroscopy: The Journal of Arthroscopic & Related Official Publication of the Arthroscopy Association North America and the International Arthroscopy Association. 2017;**33**(1):101-107

[51] Parvizi J, Pour AE, Hillibrand A, Goldberg G, Sharkey PF, Rothman RH. Back pain and Total hip arthroplasty: A prospective natural history study. Clinical Orthopaedics and Related Research. 2010;**468**(5):1325-1330

[52] Chimenti PC, Drinkwater CJ, Li W, Lemay CA, Franklin PD, O'Keefe RJ. Factors associated with early improvement in low Back pain after Total hip arthroplasty: A multi-center prospective cohort analyses. The Journal of Arthroplasty. 2016;**31**(1):176-179

[53] Okuzu Y, Goto K, Kuroda Y, Kawai T, Matsuda S. Preoperative factors associated with low Back pain improvement after Total hip arthroplasty in a Japanese population - ScienceDirect. The Journal of Arthroplasty. 2022;**37**(1):69-74

[54] Ran T, Ke S, Li J, Lyu M, Zhou Y, Zhang R, et al. Relieved low Back pain after Total hip arthroplasty in patients with both hip osteoarthritis and lumbar degenerative disease. Orthopaedic Surgery. 2021;**13**(6):1882-1889

[55] Blizzard DJ, Sheets CZ, Seyler TM, Penrose CT, Klement MR, Gallizzi MA, et al. The impact of lumbar spine disease and deformity on Total hip arthroplasty outcomes. Orthopedics. 2017;**40**(3):e520-e525

[56] Beck EC, Nwachukwu BU, Chapman R, Gowd AK, Waterman BR, Nho SJ. The influence of lumbosacral spine pathology on minimum 2-year outcome after hip arthroscopy: A nested case-control analysis. The American Journal of Sports Medicine. 2020;**48**(2):403-408

[57] Jimenez AE, Owens JS, Monahan PF, Maldonado DR, Saks BR, Sabetian PW, et al. Return to sports and minimum 2-year outcomes of hip arthroscopy in elite athletes with and without coexisting low Back pain: A propensity-matched comparison. The American Journal of Sports Medicine. 2022;**50**(1):68-78

[58] Hatem M, Martin HD. Low Back pain improves after surgery for lesser trochanteric–ischial impingement. Arthroscopy: The Journal of Arthroscopic & Related Surgery. 2021;**37**(5):1503-1509

[59] Garbuz DS, Xu M, Duncan CP, Masri BA, Sobolev B. Delays worsen quality of life outcome of primary Total

hip arthroplasty. Clinical Orthopaedics and Related Research 1976-2007. 2006;**447**:79-84

[60] Kunze KN, Beck EC, Nwachukwu BU, Ahn J, Nho SJ. Early hip arthroscopy for Femoroacetabular impingement syndrome provides superior outcomes when compared with delaying surgical treatment beyond 6 months. The American Journal of Sports Medicine. 2019;**47**(9):2038-2044

[61] Basques BA, Waterman BR, Ukwuani G, Beck EC, Neal WH, Friel NA, et al. Preoperative symptom duration is associated with outcomes after hip arthroscopy. The American Journal of Sports Medicine. 2019;**47**(1):131-137

[62] Weick J, Bawa H, Dirschl DR, Luu HH. Preoperative opioid use is associated with higher readmission and revision rates in Total knee and Total hip arthroplasty. JBJS. 2018;**100**(14):1171-1176

[63] Zusmanovich M, Thompson K, Campbell A, Youm T. Outcomes of preoperative opioid usage in hip arthroscopy: A comparison with opioid-Naïve patients. Arthroscopy: The Journal of Arthroscopic & Related Surgery. 2020;**36**(11):2832-2839.e1

[64] Nazzal EM, Wilson JM, Farley KX, Schwartz AM, Xerogeanes JW. Association of Preoperative Opioid use with Complication Rates and Resource use in patients undergoing hip arthroscopy for Femoroacetabular impingement. Orthopaedic Journal of Sports Medicine. 2021;**9**(11):23259671211045950

[65] Loth FL, Giesinger JM, Giesinger K, MacDonald DJ, Simpson AHRW, Howie CR, et al. Impact of comorbidities on outcome after Total hip arthroplasty. The Journal of Arthroplasty. 2017;**32**(9):2755-2761

[66] Mannion AF, Nauer S, Arsoy D, Impellizzeri FM, Leunig M. The association between comorbidity and the risks and early benefits of Total hip arthroplasty for hip osteoarthritis. The Journal of Arthroplasty. 2020;**35**(9):2480-2487

[67] Perets I, Chaharbakhshi EO, Barkay G, Mu BH, Lall AC, Domb BG. Diabetes mellitus is not a negative prognostic factor for patients undergoing hip arthroscopy. Orthopedics. 2021;**44**(4):241-248

[68] Sochacki KR, Brown L, Cenkus K, Di Stasi S, Harris JD, Ellis TJ. Preoperative depression is negatively associated with function and predicts poorer outcomes after hip arthroscopy for Femoroacetabular impingement. Arthroscopy: The Journal of Arthroscopic & Related Official Publication of the Arthroscopy Association North America and the International Arthroscopy Association. 2018;**34**(8):2368-2374

[69] Martin RL, Christoforetti JJ, McGovern R, Kivlan BR, Wolff AB, Nho SJ, et al. The impact of depression on patient outcomes in hip arthroscopic surgery. Orthopaedic Journal of Sports Medicine. 2018;**6**(11):2325967118806490

[70] Buller LT, Best MJ, Klika AK, Barsoum WK. The influence of psychiatric comorbidity on perioperative outcomes following primary Total hip and knee arthroplasty; a 17-year analysis of the National Hospital Discharge Survey Database. The Journal of Arthroplasty. 2015;**30**(2):165-170

Chapter 4

Diagnosis of Developmental Dysplasia of the Hip in Newborns and Infants

Nicolás Padilla-Raygoza, Gilberto Flores-Vargas, María de Jesús Gallardo-Luna, Efraín Navarro-Olivos, Marissa Padilla-Morales and Francisco J. Magos-Vázquez

Abstract

It is a review of epidemiology data of development dysplasia of the hip; it was reviewed the pre pathogenic period: agent, host and environment and the role of risk factors for the presence of developmental dysplasia of the hip. What are the clinical data for the diagnosis; the sound transmission tests for the diagnosis of the developmental dysplasia of the hip. Also, the imaging procedures for the diagnosis of the same pathology.

Keywords: dysplasia, subluxation, dislocation, clinical procedures, newborns, infant, ultrasonography

1. Introduction

The developmental dysplasia of the hip (DDH) includes a wide spectrum of abnormalities of the acetabulum and the proximal femur, including dysplasia, subluxation and dislocation of the femoral head [1–5].

In dysplasia, there is an inadequate development of the acetabulum, the femoral head or both, although there is also a concentric relationship between the 2 articular surfaces. However, in subluxated hips, although there is contact between both articular surfaces, the femoral head is not centered on the acetabular cavity [6]; in the case of dislocation the femoral head is completely out of the acetabulum [7].

Early diagnosis in the first months of life, before the child can walk, is essential, since some children with DDH go unnoticed, despite having used the usual clinical procedures, which only diagnose subluxation or dislocation, and when starting ambulation, the hip joint is injured and cannot be treated with orthopedic measures, and may lead to surgical repair of the joint; In extreme cases, the femoral head becomes necrotic, which requires the placement of a prosthesis.

2. Epidemiology and classification

It is considered that DDH occur 1 per 100 births as instability and 1 per 1000 births as subluxation or dislocation in the United States of America [8]. In Mexico, it is estimated that 1% of neonates have dysplasia and up to 75% of macrosomic neonates have hip alterations demonstrable by ultrasound, but only evolve to dislocation 1 for every 7000 live births [9].

There have been births of children with DDH, anomaly with pathological changes in the size, shape, and cellular organization of the hip that is manifested in the tissue components, soft or hard [10], which for their study are classified in CDD: typical and teratological.

The teratological is an alteration of the embryonic hip, it is called rigid, and the femoral head is outside the acetabulum and its treatment is surgical [11].

The typical or lax DDH is classified as physiological immaturity, subluxation, or dislocation, since it integrates anatomical abnormalities that affect the coxofemoral joint of children, including the abnormal edge of the acetabulum and the malposition of the femoral head causing subluxation or dislocation that affects the development of the hip before and after of birth [12–14].

This is how, within this spectrum, the defects vary from a slight difference between the articular surfaces of the iliac and femur, to the most severe case when the femoral head is outside the acetabulum; all accompanied by loss of mobility of the affected joint. So, these alterations in the hip cause disability in the infant of great social burden, especially if the child already wanders and the treatment has not been implemented properly [15].

It is important the early diagnosis, mainly before the children walk and ideally before 6 months old; if the children walk, can complicate the treatment of the DDH, and from a conservative treatment (Pavlik Harness or Fredjka Cushion), it should be surgical, with threatening prognosis for hip function.

3. Risk factors

The risk factors can be classified according to the pre- pathogenic period of the natural history of the disease, in agent, host and environment; those of the environment can be classified in microenvironment, Environment maternal and macroenvironment.

3.1 Agent

3.1.1 Maternal hormones

Relaxin is a pregnancy hormone, 6-kDa polypeptide, which increases the secretion of collagenase and activator of plasminogen, involved in collagenolysis [16]. It has been suggested that ligamentous hyperlaxity is a risk factor and that its potential to develop DC is increased due to maternal hormones such as relaxin, which are prepared prenatally to the mother's ligaments at the time of delivery [17] and cause a decrease in resistance. to the traction [11].

There are two hypotheses in relation to relaxin and DDH:

- The first is a direct effect on the laxity of fetal ligaments, since it influences the metabolism of the connective tissue by estrogen and progesterone. Higher plasma relaxin levels have been reported in dogs with DDH [18] and cord blood from babies with DDH, although the differences were not statistically significant [19].

- Another hypothesis suggests that low concentrations of relaxin are associated with DDH, since in the absence of sufficient laxity of the maternal ligaments, there will be greater pressure on the fetus and may originate DDH [20–22].

3.2 Host

3.2.1 Heritage

It is considered that there is influence of multifactorial inheritance, combining genetics and environmental conditions; 20% of cases have a family history, 6% if one of the parents was affected, 12% if it was one of the parents and a brother and 37% in monozygotic twins. Up to 20% of these cases have been associated with congenital malformations, such as clubfoot, amniotic bands of the pelvic limbs and congenital muscular torticollis [17]. Ömeroğlu et al., reported in a retrospective study, that there was an association of having a family history of CD with presenting DDH compared with infants who did not have DDH (P = .02, OR = 2.10) [23], although Mendoza et al., in Mexican neonates, found no statistical association between family history of DDHC and DDH in the neonate (P = .73, OR = 0.83) [24].

3.2.2 Position in utero

The breech presentation, especially with the pelvic extremities in extension and adduction, have been indicated as risk factors for DC as well as for hip dislocation since it occurs in 30–50% of cases [10]. Ömeroğlu et al., Reported that breech presentation is associated with DC (P = .015, OR = 1.87) [23]. In the study of Mexican children, a strong statistical association was reported between breech presentation and DC (P =, 004, OR = 5.32] [24].

3.2.3 Firstborn

Being the first child, the uterine force will be greater, being able to exert greater tension to the product [17]. Ömeroğlu et al., studied the relationship with female first-born and DDH; they did not find no association with DDH [23].

3.2.4 Ethnicity

It is considered that the frequency of DC in white race is of 50: 1 compared with African race; it is more frequent among American Indians and Eskimos than in South American or African Indians [11]. Eskimos and American Indians overdress children with legs in extension and adduction or move them in wooden strollers with narrow space; The Huichols in Mexico transport their babies in their body by hanging their limbs in abduction [11]. Highest incidence were reported from Finland, Croatia and Canada (5–195 per 1000), with very low incidences among populations in sub-Saharan Africa and Hong Kong (0–0.1 per 1000) [25]. Geographical and cultural factors regarding climate differences and the practice of swaddling respectively may in part explain this variation [26, 27].

3.2.5 Female sex

It has been reported that the frequency of hip dislocation is more common among women (7:1) in relation to men [11], but DDH is more common in men with up to 1% of live new-borns. Ömeroğlu et al., reported no association between female gender and DDH [23].

3.2.6 High birth weight

In a series of 100 macrosomic neonates in Celaya, Mexico, Figueroa et al., reported that 100% of neonates with clinical maneuvers suggestive of DDH, had ultrasonographic data of DDH and 75% of those with clinical maneuvers negatives, also presented ultrasonographic data of DDH [9].

3.3 Environment

3.3.1 Microenvironment

3.3.1.1 Oligohydramnios

The presence of little amniotic fluid has been indicated as a risk factor for DDH [11, 17], but Ömeroğlu et al., in Turkey, in a retrospective study, found no association between oligohydramnios and DDH in children with DDH compared with children with healthy hips [23]. It is assumed that having little amniotic fluid the contraction force of the uterus will be greater and will affect the product; It is also suggested that by decreasing the amniotic fluid, the product will have more space to place their pelvic extremities in extension and adduction, favoring the instability of the hip.

3.3.1.2 Breech presentation

The breech presentation has been implicated as a risk factor in DDH [4]; products with breech presentation, have twice the risk of DDH [23], the risk is strengthened if it is with the pelvic extremities in extension and intrauterine adduction [10]. Another mechanism is the traction of the pelvic extremities, exerting pressure on the hips for the extraction of a product with breech presentation [11].

3.3.2 Environment maternal

3.3.2.1 Primiparous

The idea that primiparous women have a greater risk of having offspring with DDH due to greater strength of the uterine musculature has been strengthened, which upon contracting will generate greater pressure in the product, but possibly also, due to the fact of a narrower intrauterine cavity [11].

3.3.2.2 Nutrition

Maternal alcoholism has been invoked as a risk factor for DDH [11, 15] and in canine animal models, some dietary factors that favor DDH and the severity of it have been reported [16]. Excessive caloric intake leads to rapid growth and early overload of the bone system and causes an increase in the frequency and severity of DDH in genetically susceptible dogs during the first 6 months of life [16, 28].

It has also been pointed out that elevated serum levels of vitamin C could decrease the frequency of DDH [16], but controlled studies could not demonstrate this [29]. Excessive consumption of vitamin D increases intestinal absorption and renal calcium reabsorption, and this may increase the risk of DDH in canine models [16]. This has led to a tendency to increase the frequency of DDH in the cold months [30–32] but this does not happen in Finland where the highest frequency was in the months of June and July [33].

Smoking has also been reported as a risk factor for DDH [16].

3.3.3 Macroenvironment

3.3.3.1 Swaddling or excessive clothing

Excessive clothing has been reported as a risk factor in DDH [9, 11]; Mendoza-Lara et al., reported a strong association ($P < 0.0004$) of swaddling with the pelvic extremities in extension and adduction, with DDH [24]. This has led to a tendency to increase the frequency of DDH in the cold months [30–32] but this does not happen in Finland where the highest frequency was in the months of June and July [33].

3.3.3.2 Pull on the hip

Obstetric trauma, traction on the hips to extract a product in breech presentation, hold the neonate, after birth, of the heels without support in the back, can cause elongation of the ligaments of the hip and cause DDH [11, 16].

4. Clinical diagnosis

If DDH is in a newborn or children, before to walk, clinical maneuvers as Ortolani, Barlow, Peter-Baden, piston, limitation of abduction can detect, only subluxation or dislocation of the hip. Dysplasia is not detected by these maneuvers.

The sound transmission tests can detect dysplasia, subluxation or dislocation [34–37].

From the neonatal stage to one year of age, at each visit to the health worker, the following clinical maneuvers should be intentionally sought according to the type of pathology.

4.1 Ortolani's sign

It is found in subluxable lax hips and is absent in teratological (**Figure 1**) [17]. Both extremities are taken, one in each hand, placing the knees between the thumb and forefinger, flexing the hips up to 90°, and resting the palm of the hand on the flexed

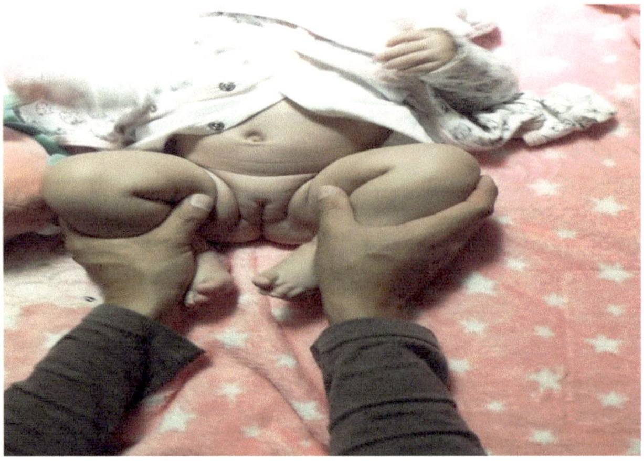

Figure 1.
Ortolani sign.

knee and the fingers along the femur, with the Point of the third finger on the greater trochanter, fix the opposite hip by applying slight pressure of the knee towards the table. The hip under examination is pressed vertically and gentle adduction abduction movements are made, looking for the click that occurs when the femoral head jumps over the cartilaginous labrum.

4.2 Barlow's sign

It detects subluxation or dislocation hips, the side to be explored is taken with the hand along the femur, with the middle finger located on the greater trochanter and the

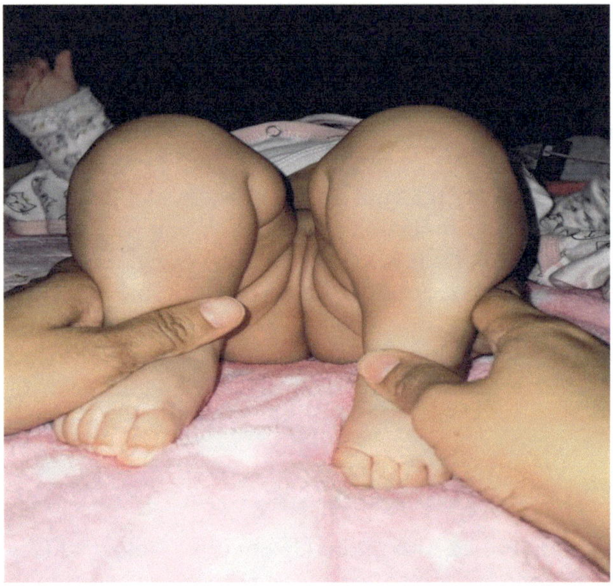

Figure 2.
Galeazzi sign.

thumb on the lesser trochanter [17]; hip flexion 90° and abducted 45°; with the other hand the pelvis is fixed. Femur movements are made from front to back. It is considered positive when abnormal play is perceived, and the femoral head moves anteroposteriorly. It occurs in 75% of newborns but disappears after 30 days in 85% of them.

4.3 Galeazzi sign

The patient is placed supine with the hips and knees bent and the feet resting in the plane of the examination table, observing the difference in height of the knees (**Figure 2**) [17]. The problem side is lowered compared to the opposite side.

4.4 Dupuytren's sign or piston

The patient is placed supine with the leg flexed to 90° at the hip and knee [17]. The pelvis is fixed with the thumb of one hand resting on the anterior superior iliac spine and the index and middle fingers on the trochanter; With the other hand he takes the knee and the leg, making movements up and down (traction and pressure). If it is positive, the displacement of the greater trochanter is perceived.

4.5 Sign of abduction limitation

Patient in supine position, with 90° flexion in hips and knees, gently abducting both legs at the same time [17]. The affected side will show limited abduction. Newborns are abducted at 90°; at 15 days of birth it is 60–70°.

4.6 Peter-Baden sign or fold asymmetry

It is the asymmetry and increase in the number of the inguinal and gluteal folds; in general, the affected side shows higher folds than the opposite limb (**Figure 3**) [17].

4.7 Comparative sound transmission test with tuning fork and stethoscope

The patient is placed supine with the lower extremities in extension and adduction; a 256-cycle/second tuning fork is placed on one knee and the sound is captured through a stethoscope, placing the diaphragm on the symphysis pubis; the tuning fork is placed on the opposite knee and the sound is compared to the first side (**Figure 4a** and **b**) [34–37]. If the sound is less on either side, it is considered positive for that side. If the DDC is bilateral, the perception of sound will be the same on both sides.

4.8 Sound transmission test with extension/flexion

The patient is placed supine and the pelvic limbs are aligned in extension and adduction; the tuning fork is placed on one knee and the stethoscope with its diaphragm is placed on the symphysis pubis; sound is captured; the knee and hip are flexed to 90° and the sound is perceived; it is considered positive if the bending sound increases, if it decreases or stays the same, it is considered negative (**Figure 5**) [34–37].

For the extension/flexion sound transmission test, the neonate is placed supine with the lower extremities in extension and adduction; the tuning fork is placed on the knee on one side and the stethoscope is placed on the symphysis pubis and the sound is perceived; the hip and knee are flexed to 90° and the sound is perceived: if

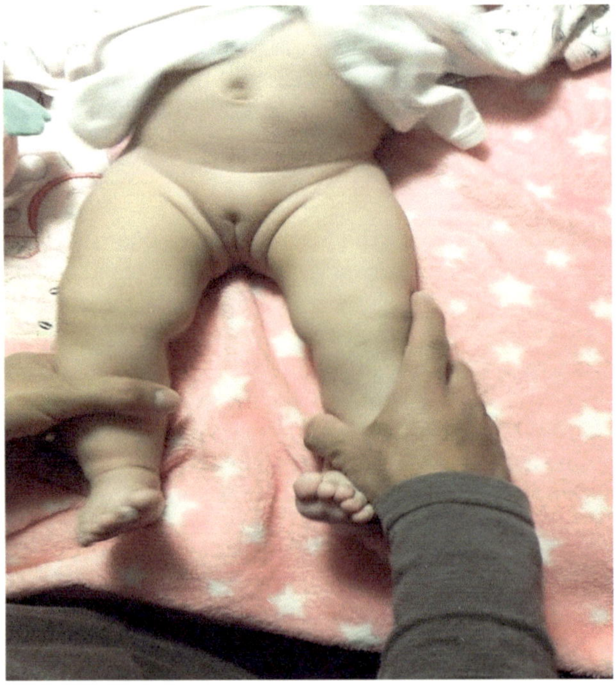

Figure 3.
Peter-Baden sign.

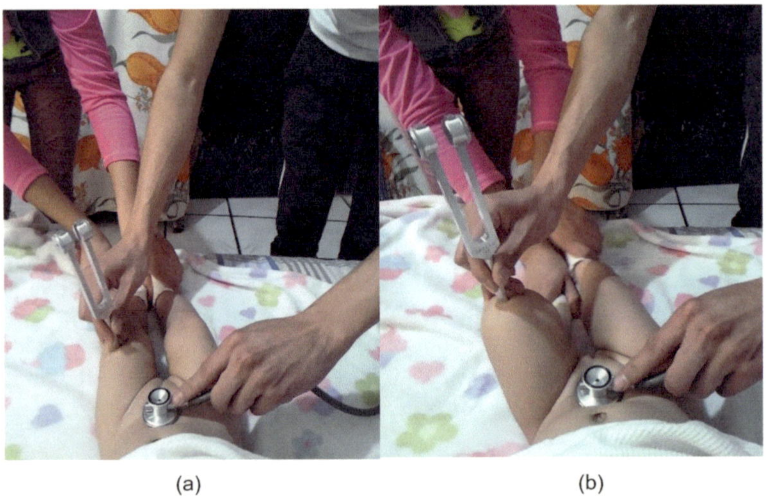

Figure 4.
a. Compared sound transmission. b. Sound transmission with extension/flexion.

the sound is lower or equal, the hip is healthy, if the sound increase, the hip has DDH. The opposite side is subsequently evaluated [34–37].

Sound transmission test with bone radar ® (University of Guanajuato, Mexico) or electroacoustic probe (Patent pending, University of Guanajuato) [35, 36].

Starting from the properties of bone to transmit sound, we developed a device to apply sound transmission tests in an objective way. The device consists of a sound

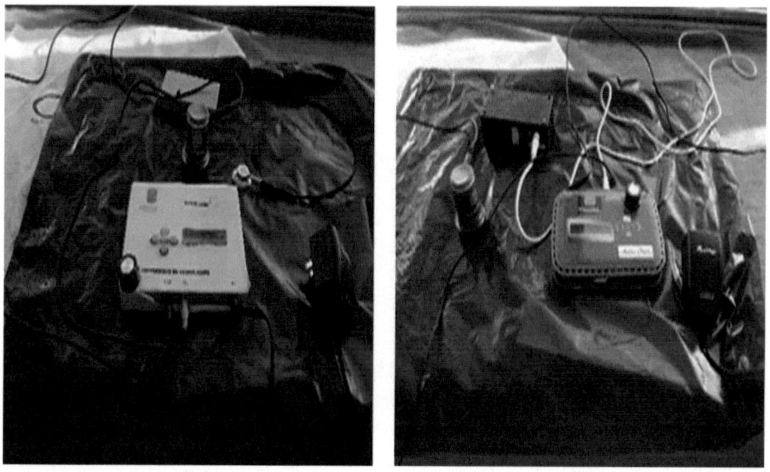

(a) (b)

Figure 5.
The above figures are using device in flexion of the hip.

generator, a receiver placed on a stethoscope and a screen where the sound waves appear transformed into digits [35–37].

For the comparative sound transmission test, the newborn is placed supine with the pelvic limbs in extension and adduction; the sound generator is placed on the knee on one side and the receiver on the symphysis pubis, the digits are recorded on screens; the sound generator is placed on the opposite knee and the digits are recorded on the screen. If there is a difference in the numbers on either side, it is considered positive. In cases of bilateral CDD, the record will be the same on both sides [34–37].

For the extension/flexion sound transmission test, the neonate is placed supine with the lower extremities in extension and adduction; the sound generator is placed on the knee on one side and the receiver is placed on the symphysis pubis and the digits are recorded on the screen; the hip and knee are flexed to 90° and the digits are recorded on the screen; If the digits on the screen are greater in flexion than in extension, it is considered positive. The opposite side is subsequently evaluated [34–37].

For sound transmission test with electroacoustic probe, the technique is the same that bone radar ®, only the digits in screen are decibels.

4.9 Complementary clinical diagnosis

When the child is walking, look for the Trendelenburg and Duchenne signs. Older children who are already wandering, with undiagnosed CDD, present claudication, duck gait (in bilateral cases), increased lumbar lordosis, toe gait, and a discrepancy in the length of the lower extremities.

5. Complications

Recurrent dislocation, avascular necrosis of the femoral head, femoral fracture, and nerve palsy are the most common. The most fearsome complication is avascular necrosis of the femoral head, which is due to the reduction, producing cartilaginous compression and occlusion of extraosseous and intra-articular epiphyseal vessels, causing partial or total necrosis of the femoral head.

6. Diagnostic imaging

Diagnosis in the newborn is clinical and is made through the hereditarily and perinatal antecedents, as well as by the maneuvers of the deliberate exploration. In case of doubt, an echo-sonogram of the hip is used by qualified imaging specialists; It should be noted that radiographs are not useful before 4 months of extrauterine life.

Ultrasonographic diagnosis is made in the newborn and at any other stage of life; It is performed through the static and dynamic test of the hip, with the Graf technique, where the angles α and β are measured in each test. Graph I is considered a normal hip in the child with $\alpha > 60°$ and $\beta < 55°$; Graf II is considered a physiologically immature hip with α 44–59° and β 55–77°; Graph III and IV as a dislocated or dislocated hip with $\alpha < 43°$ and $\beta > 77°$ (**Figure 6a b**) [38, 39].

The radiological diagnosis is based on the findings of the anteroposterior pelvic plates in neutral position and abducted 45° (Lowestein position). The study is useful from the fourth month of age, since the ossification nuclei of the femoral head have already appeared. The following radiographic data can be found: Hilgenrainer's line is a horizontal one that passes through the triradial cartilages of the iliac; the Perkins or Ombredanne line is a vertical line that passes perpendicularly through the outermost edge of the acetabulum until it surpasses the Hilgenreiner line, forming the Putti quadrants (the femoral head must be in the lower inner quadrant, normally). The angle formed with line that start from the outer edge of the acetabulum and pass through the bottom of the acetabulum until reaching Hilgenreiner line, and Hilgenreiner line, gives us the acetabular index that must be less than 30° (**Figure 7a**) [11, 17].

The Shenton's arch, passes through the lower edge of the pubis and continues with the lower edge of the femoral neck, forming a normal arch; if there is distortion of this arch, it is considered a dislocated hip (**Figure 7a**) [11, 17].

Figure 7 a represents the anteroposterior plate of the pelvis in abduction; Look for the Von Rossen sign by drawing a line along the axis of the femur to the midline of the spine (King's midline); the line usually passes through the acetabulum [11, 17].

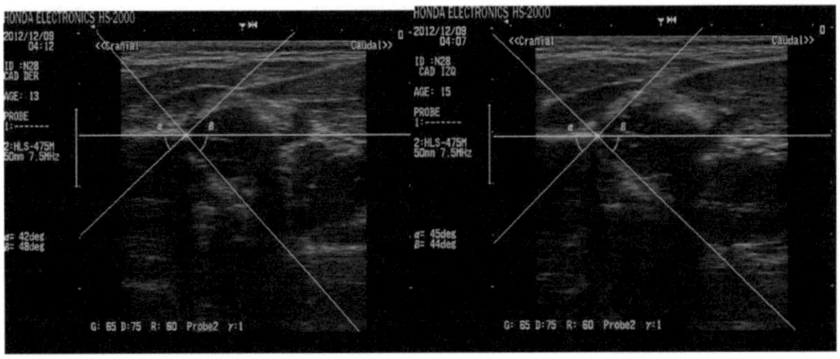

(a) (b)

Figure 6.
a. Graf technique left hip. b. Graf technique right hip.

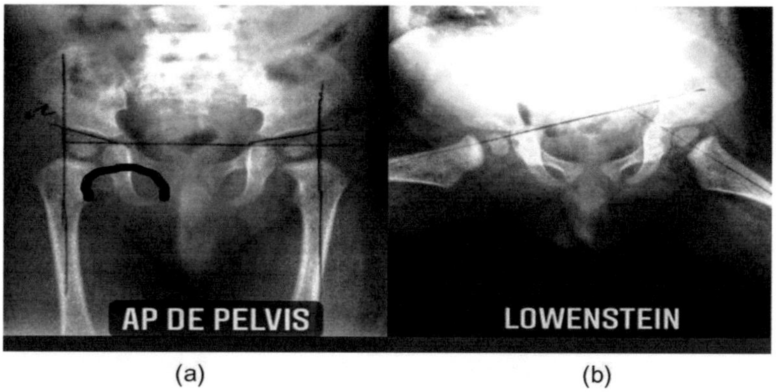

Figure 7.
a. AP of the hip. b. Lowenstein. Source: Dr. Jaime González-García.

Diagnosis at an early stage (under 2 months): in the dislocated hip there is an increase in the acetabular index and absence of the peak of the acetabulum eyebrow. In the dislocated and subluxed hip, lateralization of the proximal internal end of the neck, Von Rossen sign, and alteration of Shenton's line are located [11, 17].

Late stage diagnosis: in addition to the above, there is Putti's triad (increased acetabular index, the proximal end of the femur outside and above the Perkins line, as well as delayed ossification of the nucleus of the femoral head) [11, 17].

7. Treatment

Treatment will depend on the age at which the diagnosis is made; the best prognosis is obtained at the beginning of the management in the newborn. In teratological dislocation, the management will always be surgical. In the subluxable hip, wide and thick cushions are used to maintain abduction of the hips bilaterally; they are used for a time in months that is calculated by multiplying the age in months by two when making the diagnosis; monthly clinical control should be performed. Recommending the use of a double diaper should be avoided, because disposable diapers do not maintain hip abduction [11, 17].

In the dislocated and dislocated hip, the abduction of the thighs is achieved, giving stability to the hips, with the use of the Pavlik harness, Fredjka cushion, Von Rossen splint, Barlow splint; These devices remain in place until a stronger joint capsule is obtained, which is achieved in 3 to 6 months.

If the child is already walking and the hip problem has not been detected, the treatment can be surgical and in severe cases, in the event of necrosis of the femoral head, place a prosthesis.

8. Discussion

When receiving a newborn, a checklist for risk factors should be applied, already indicated as suggested by Ömeroğlu et al. [23], and if the infant has one or more, should undergo a Graf ultrasound of the hips to establish whether there is a diagnosis of DDH. The use of clinical tests such as Ortolani, Barlow and others should be postponed until the fourth day of extrauterine life, since there will be false positives due to the processes of Birth, such as passage through the birth canal or potentially the effects of relaxin.

From the fourth day of life, comparative sound transmission tests can be applied, which have shown good sensitivity compared to hip ultrasound [12, 13, 35–37], unlike the usual clinical maneuvers that show low sensitivity for DDH [13, 35, 37].

Why to use sound transmission tests? **Table 1** show validity of the sound transmission test and sound transmission test with extension/flexion.

The compared sound transmission test evaluate both hips, if them have dysplasia, the test give a false negative; this is avoid using the compared sound transmission test with extension/flexion,

It was reported, sensitivity for Ortolani de 5.11%, specificity 96.77%, positive predictive value 69.23%, and negative predictive value 41.81% [13].

For Barlow test, Padilla et al. [13] reported 2.27, 99.19, 80.00, and 41.69%, respectively.

For repeatability, Padilla et al. [35] reported Kappa 0.80 intra-observer and 0.70 inter-observer, for compared sound transmission test and, Kappa.88 and 0.78, intra-observer and inter-observer, respectively, for the sound transmission test with extension/flexion.

With electroacoustic probe, the repeatability was Kappa 0.80 intra-observer and 0.81 inter-observer for compared sound transmission; 0,98 intra. Observer and 0.95 inter-observer, for compared sound transmission with extension/flexion [37].

Since the 80's of the 20th century, the use of ultrasound of the hips has been recommended instead of radiographs in the newborn and in infants less than 8 weeks of extrauterine life, since with radiography, diagnostic errors are generated due to the lack of ossification of the femoral head mainly.

If the presence of DDH is adequately orthopedically treated, the cure is complete with an excellent prognosis, and this is darkened if it comes to surgical treatment.

	Sensibility	Specifity	Positive predictive value	Negative predictive value
Comparative sound transmission				
Padilla et al. [12] Padilla et al. [13]	72.7	86.6	NR	NR
Padilla et al. [35] Padilla et al. [37]	27.7	94.35	87.27	47.7
	60.9	92	51.9	95
	44.83	97.66	76.47	91.26
	37.93	98.83	84.62	90.37
	37.93	97.66	73.33	90.27
Comparative sound transmission with extension/flexion				
Padilla et al. [12]	74.4	96.9	NR	NR
Padilla et al. [13]	86.36	87.09	90.47	81.81
Padilla et al. [35]	82.6	96.2	73.1	97.8
Padilla et al. [37]	82.76	99.42	96.00	97.14
	82.76	100.0	100.0	97.16
	86.21	100.0	100.0	97.71

Table 1.
Validity of the sound transmission tests.

In infants, DDH is treated with a Fredjka cushion or Pavlik harness; the double diaper should not be used; if the child is already ambulant, he should be evaluated for surgical treatment of the hip joint. And in this phase, the presence of necrosis of the femoral head should be assessed, since this will lead to the placement of a prosthesis.

The objective of diagnosis and treatment is that the child does not reach the stage of ambulation with DDH and avoid surgical treatment, which is a major procedure.

9. Conclusion

It is a pathology that can go unnoticed and its best prognosis is to detect and treat it before 6 months of age.

The health professional in charge of the care of neonates and infants, should be attentive at each visit, of the state of the hips of each child, applying the usual clinical maneuvers and sound transmission tests, and, if necessary, ultrasound of the hips, and with this, is possible to establish an early diagnostic of DDH.

The objective is to avoid that infants suffer corrective surgery of the hip and/or replacement of the hip.

Acknowledgements

Not funding for this manuscript.

Conflict of interest

Nothing to declare.

Ethics for images

The parents from children give their consent to publish the images because the children cannot be identify.

Author details

Nicolás Padilla-Raygoza[1*], Gilberto Flores-Vargas[1], María de Jesús Gallardo-Luna[1], Efraín Navarro-Olivos[2], Marissa Padilla-Morales[3] and Francisco J. Magos-Vázquez[4]

1 Department of Research and Technological Development, Directorate of Teaching and Research, Institute of Public Health from Guanajuato State, Guanajuato, México

2 Directorate of Teaching and Research, Institute of Public Health from Guanajuato State, Guanajuato, México

3 Division of Health Sciences and Engineering, Campus Celaya-Salvatierra, University of Guanajuato, Celaya, México

4 Directorate of Health Services, Institute of Public Health from Guanajuato State, Guanajuato, México

*Address all correspondence to: npadillar@guanajuato.gob.mx

References

[1] Dezateux C, Rosendahl K. Developmental dysplasia of the hip. Lancet. 2007;**369**:1541-1552. DOI: 10.1016/S0140-6736(07)60710-7

[2] Dunn PM. The anatomy and pathology of congenital dislocation of the hip. Clinical Orthopaedics and Related Research. 1976;**119**:23-27

[3] Ponseti IV. Morphology of the acetabulum in congenital dislocation of the hip. Gross, histological and roentgenographic studies. The Journal of Bone and Joint Surgery. American Volume. 1978;**60**:586-599

[4] Lee MC, Eberson CP. Growth and development of the child's hip. The Orthopedic Clinics of North America. 2006;**37**:119-132. DOI: 10.1016/j.ocl.2005.12.001

[5] Noordin S, Umer M, Hafeez K, Nawaz H. Developmental dysplasia of the hip. Orthopedic Reviews. 2010;**2**:e19. DOI: 10.4081/or.2010.e19

[6] Weinstein SL. Congenital hip dislocation. Long-range problems, residual signs, and symptoms after successful treatment. Clinical Orthopaedics and Related Research. 1992;**281**:69-74

[7] Wiberg G. Shelf operation in congenital dysplasia of the acetabulum and in subluxation and dislocation of the hip. The Journal of Bone and Joint Surgery. American Volume. 1953;**35ª**:65-80

[8] American Academy of Pediatrics. Committee of Quality Improvement. Subcommittee on developmental dysplasia of the hip. Pediatrics. 2000; **105**:896-905

[9] Figueroa Ferrari RC, Padilla-Raygoza N. La luxación congénita de cadera en el recién nacido macrosómico Aspectos ultrasonográficos. Rev. Med. IMSS (Mex). 1994;**32**:277-279

[10] Pruszczynski B, Harcke HT, Holmes L, Bowen JR. Natural history of hip instability in infants (without subluxation or dislocation): A three year follow-up. BMC Musculoskeletal Disorders. 2014;**2014**(15):355. DOI: 10.1186/1471-247415-355

[11] Padilla-Raygoza N. Displasia congénita de cadera. Historia natural y niveles de prevención. Revista Mexicana de Pediatría. 1991;**58**(6):337-345

[12] Padilla-Raygoza N, Figueroa-Ferrari RC. Diagnóstico de la luxación congénita de cadera mediante la transmisión comparada del sonido. Revista Mexicana de Pediatría. 1992;**59**(5):149-151

[13] Padilla-Raygoza N, Figueroa-Ferrari RC. Pruebas de transmisión del sonido en el diagnóstico de la luxación congénita de cadera en el neonato. Revista Mexicana de Pediatría. 1996;**63**(6):265-268

[14] Secretaria de Salud. Guía Clínica Preventiva Diagnóstico y tratamiento oportuno de la displasia en el desarrollo de cadera. 2013. Available from: http://www.cenetec.salud.gob.mx/descargas/gpc/CatalogoMaestro/091_GPC_Displasiacaderaped/SSA_091_08_EyR.pdf

[15] Cymet J, Alvarez MM, García G, Frías R, Meza A, Rosales ME, et al. El diagnóstico oportuno de la displasia de la cadera. Enfermedad discapacitante de por vida. Consenso del Colegio

Mexicano de Ortopedia y Traumatología. Acta Ortopédica Mexicana. 2011, 2011;**25**(5):313-322 Available from: http://www.medigraphic.com/pdfs/ortope/or-2011/or115j.pdf

[16] Rhodes AML, Clarke NMP. A review of environmental factors implicated in human developmental dysplasia of the hip. Journal of Children's Orthopaedics. 2014;**8**:375-379. DOI: 10.1007/s11832-014-0615-y

[17] Padilla-Raygoza N. Displasia del desarrollo de la cadera (Luxación congénita de cadera). En: Martínez y Martínez R, ed. La salud del niño y del adolescente. 8ª ed., México, D.F., El Manual Moderno, Vol. II, 2018

[18] Goldsmith L, Lust G, Steinetz B. Transmission of relaxin from lactating bitches to their offspring via suckling. Biology of Reproduction. 1994;**50**:258-265

[19] Borthwick GM, Borthwick AC, Grant P, Mac Lennan AH. Relaxin levels in the human: An indicator of target, storage and production sites. In: Mac Lennan AH, Tregear GW, Bryant Greenwood GD, editors. Progress in Relaxin Research. Singapore: World Scientific Publishing Co.; 1995. pp. 25-60

[20] Forst J, Forst C, Forst R, et al. Pathogenetic relevance of the pregnancy hormone relaxin to inborn hip instability. Archives of Orthopaedic and Trauma Surgery. 1997;**116**:209-212

[21] Dunn P. Congenital postural deformities: Further perinatal associations. Proceedings of the Royal Society of Medicine. 1974;**67**:32-36

[22] Dunn P. Perinatal observations on the etiology of congenital dislocation of the hip. Clinical Orthopaedics. 1976;**119**:11-22

[23] Ömeroglu H, Akceylan A, Köse N. Associations between risk factors and developmental dysplasia of the hip and ultrasonographic hip type: A retrospective case control study. Journal of Children's Orthopaedics. 2019;**13**:161-166. DOI: 10.1302/1863-2548.13.180174

[24] Mendoza-Lara C, Padilla-Raygoza N, Olvera-Villanueva G, Delgado-Sandoval SC. Risk factor for developmental dysplasia of the hip in new-borns from Celaya, Guanajuato, Mexico: A cross-sectional study. BJMMR. 2016;**12**(10):1-7. DOI: 10.9734/BJMMR/2016/23125

[25] Mitchell P, Redfern R. The prevalence of dislocation in developmental dysplasia of the hip in britain over the past 1,000 years. Journal of Pediatric Orthopedics. 2007;**27**(8):890-892. DOI: 10.1097/bpo.0b013e31815a6091

[26] Kutlu A, Memik R, Mutlu M, et al. Congenital dislocation of the hip and its relation to swaddling used in Turkey. Journal of Pediatric Orthopedics. 1992;**12**(5):598-602

[27] Kremli MK, Alshahid AH, Khoshhal KI, Zamzam MM. The pattern of developmental dysplasia of the hip. Saudi Medical Journal. 2003;**24**(10):1118-1120

[28] Fries C, Remedios A. The pathogenesis and diagnosis of canine hip dysplasia: A review. The Canadian Veterinary Journal. 1995;**36**:494-502

[29] Bennett D. Hip dysplasia and ascorbate therapy: Fact or fancy? Seminars in Veterinary Medicine and Surgery (Small Animal). 1987;**2**:152-157

[30] Anand JK, Moden I, Myles JW. Incidence of neonatal hip instability: Are there seasonal variations? Acta

Orthopaedica Belgica. 1992;**58**(2): 205-208

[31] Valdivieso Garcia JL, Blanco Lopez F, Ocana Losa LM, Romanos LA. Seasonal incidence of congenital hip dislocation. A risk factor. Anales Españoles de Pediatría. 1989;**31**(6):567-569

[32] Aguirre-Negrete MG, Garcia de Alba-Garcia JE, Ramirez-Soltero SE. Congenital hip dislocation and the seasons. Boletín Médico del Hospital Infantil de México. 1991;**48**(4):243-248

[33] Heikkila E. Congenital dislocation of the hip in Finland. An epidemiologic analysis of 1,035 cases. Acta Orthopaedica Scandinavica. 1984;**55**(2):125-129. DOI: 10.3109/17453678408992322

[34] Stone M, Richardson J, Bennet G. Another clinical test for congenital dislocation of the hip. Lancet. 1987;**1**:954-955

[35] Padilla-Raygoza N, Diaz-Guerrero R, Ruiz-Paloalto ML, Córdova-Fraga T, Sosa-Aquino MA, Perez-Oliva HA. Validity and reliability of a measuring device basedon sound transmission for diagnosis of hip displasia in newborns. Advances in Bioscience and Biotechnology. 2014;**5**:831-837. DOI: 10.4236/abb.2014.510097

[36] Padilla-Raygoza N, Medina-Alvarez D, Ruiz-Paloalto ML, Cordova-Fraga T, Sosa-Aquino MA, Perez-Olivas AH. Diagnosis of developmental displasia of the hip using sound transmission inneonates. Health. 2014;**6**:2510-2516. DOI: 10.4236/health.2014.618289

[37] Padilla-Raygoza N, Olvera-Villanueva G, Delgado-Sandoval MC, Córdova-Fraga T, Sosa-Aquino MA, Beltrán-Campos V. Validity and reliability of electroacoustic probe for diagnosis of developmental dysplasia of the hip. BMC Pediatrics. 2017;**17**:149. DOI: 10.1186/s12887-017-0903-z

[38] Arti H, Mehdinasab SA, Arti S. Comparing results of clinical versus ultrasonographic examination in developmental dysplasia of hip. Journal of Research in Medical Sciences. 2013;**18**(12):1051-1055

[39] Kowalczyk B, Felus J, Kwinta P. Developmental dysplasia of the hip: The problems in the diagnosis process in our own experience. Medycyna Wieku Rozwojowego. 2005;**9**(3):395-406

Section 3

Hip Surgery

Chapter 5

The Direct Anterior Approach: A Comprehensive Guide for the Learner and Educator

Bijan Dehghani, Avi Dravid, Praneeth Thota and Neil P. Sheth

Abstract

Total hip arthroplasty is one of the most widely performed procedures demonstrating excellent clinical outcomes and implant longevity. Enhanced imaging modalities, advancements in material science, and improvements in surgical technique have contributed to the global success of this procedure. One such technique has gained significant attention over the past decade – the direct anterior approach (DAA). First described by Carl Hueter in 1881, the DAA is now more commonly credited to Smith-Peterson. This technique demonstrates rapid recovery, reduced hospital length of stay, and enhanced stability. Despite these advantages, there is a well reported learning curve for surgeons, particularly for those who trained using an alternative surgical approach. In this chapter we explore a methodological approach to mitigate and decrease the learning curve; allowing for a safe and reproducible guide to teach surgeons how to transition to the DAA.

Keywords: total hip arthroplasty, direct anterior approach, learning curve, hip replacement, posterior approach

1. Introduction

Total Hip Arthroplasty (THA) is one of the most commonly performed orthopaedic procedures for the treatment of end-stage hip degeneration. With a robust track record of effectiveness and safety, THA has become a widely accepted method for providing pain relief, restoring function, and reestablishing a patient's quality of life [1]. Sir John Charnley pioneered one of the first low friction arthroplasties in the 1950s, laying the groundwork for future advancement in the field [2]. Since then, advents in technology in the arena of biomaterials, implant design, and surgical technique have contributed to THA's widespread acceptance [1]. An estimated 370,770 hip replacements were performed in 2014, with this number expected to reach 635,000 in 2030; this represents a projected 71% increase [3]. A rapidly aging population, widening surgical indications, as well as an increased prevalence of obesity and associated osteoarthritis have fueled this increase in demand [4].

Total hip arthroplasty can be performed through several surgical exposures, including the posterior, posterolateral, direct lateral, anterolateral, and direct anterior

 IntechOpen

approaches [2]. The direct anterior approach (DAA), in particular, has exhibited a tremendous amount of enthusiasm in recent years. German surgeon Carl Hueter first characterized the anterior approach for accessing the hip joint in 1881, describing an inter-nervous and inter-muscular plane between the tensor fasciae latae and sartorius muscles – known today as the Hueter Interval [5]. However, American surgeon Marius Nygaard Smith-Petersen is credited with popularizing this surgical approach. Although this surgical approach was first adopted as a means of reducing congenital hip dislocations, Smith-Petersen also used it to perform mold arthroplasties in 1949 [2, 5].

There is a growing body of literature substantiating the benefits of the DAA. This surgical approach is considered less invasive, exhibits greater stability compared to other approaches, and results in less overall tissue damage [6, 7]. A randomized clinical study comparing the DAA and the posterior approach demonstrated lower pain scores and better function during the early stages of recovery with the DAA [8]. Additional studies have reported lower pain scores, less blood loss, and increased walking speed compared to the direct lateral approach [9]. In the immediate post-operative period, the DAA patients were discharged from the hospital earlier and with greater mobility [10]. However, other studies have shown that differences in post-operative recovery may not be clinically significant as they equalize by 6 weeks, and maintain in the longer term [6] Regardless of surgical approach, clinical success in THA is predicated on adequate surgical exposure, correct component position, and proper soft-tissue balancing [11].

Patient demand, as well as marketing by industry and orthopaedic practices has contributed to the rise in popularity of the DAA [11]. In an effort to meet demand, surgeons may choose to switch from an alternative surgical approach, but, the steep learning curve has always been a major barrier, especially if the transition occurs once already in practice and dedicated time to pursue formal fellowship training is not practical. The DAA is typically performed with the patient in a supine position, requiring different sets of retractors, and often use of a specialized operative table [12]. Some studies suggest that surgeons should perform at least 100 such operations in order to become adequately proficient in the technique [12].

Adult reconstruction fellowships and orthopaedic residency training programs have taken notice of this enthusiasm for the DAA, and have addressed this demand through formal didactics, surgical videos, hands-on training, cadaveric workshops, and educational simulation platforms [13]. For surgeons that do not have the luxury of formally training, a systematic, dedicated methodology must be employed when transitioning to the DAA in order to minimize complications, achieve favorable clinical outcomes, and recognize the benefits associated with the surgical approach.

2. Surgical technique of the direct anterior approach

The first step in learning the DAA is understanding the anatomy, and more particularly the anterior structures of the hip. The important landmarks include the anterior superior iliac spine (ASIS) and the greater trochanter (GT). Proper equipment and positioning are paramount for successful procedure. A specialized surgical table is often used to allow for controlled manipulation of the extremity; however, many surgeons successfully perform this procedure using a regular table. The Hana table is commonly described for this purpose as it allows the surgeon to apply traction, rotate, and abduct/adduct the extremity as needed. The principal author of this paper utilizes a Medacta table extension which can be readily attached to a regular surgical table. The patient is positioned supine with a triangular bump under the hip to assist with hip extension. The bump should be placed proximal 1/3 and middle 1/3 of the femur making sure that a hand can be freely moved over the bump.

The surgical incision is marked out 2 cm distal and 3 cm lateral to the ASIS (**Figure 1**); the top of the incision is typically at the midpoint between the ASIS and the tip of the GT. The superficial dissection is performed down to the level of the TFL fascia which can be identified based on the blue tint of the muscle belly deep to the fascia (**Figure 2**). Using electrocautery or a scalpel, the TFL fascia is incised in-line with the muscle fibers and carefully separated from the muscle belly. It is important to stay parallel with the muscle fibers to ensure minimal bleeding and muscle damage. Retracting the released TFL laterally completes the superficial dissection and should expose the fascial floor of the TFL. The TFL is a digastric muscle, therefore, it is critical to make sure that both muscle bellies are retracted laterally.

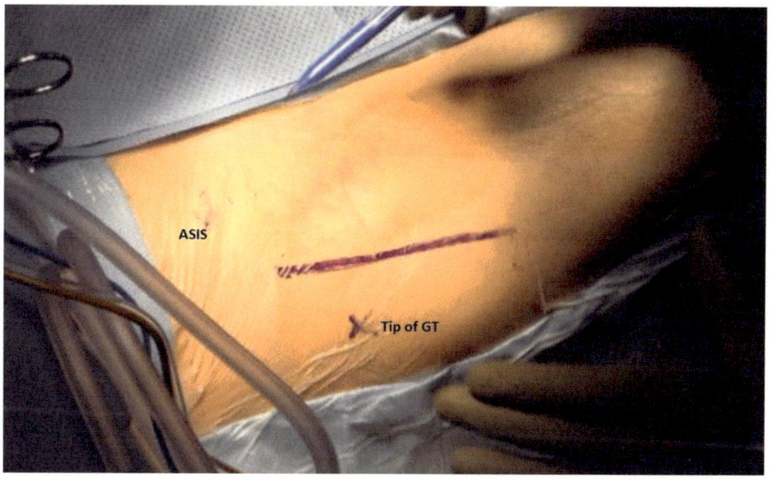

Figure 1.
Incision placement for the direct anterior approach. The trajectory of the incision follows the muscle belly of the tensor fascia latae (TFL) (Right hip).

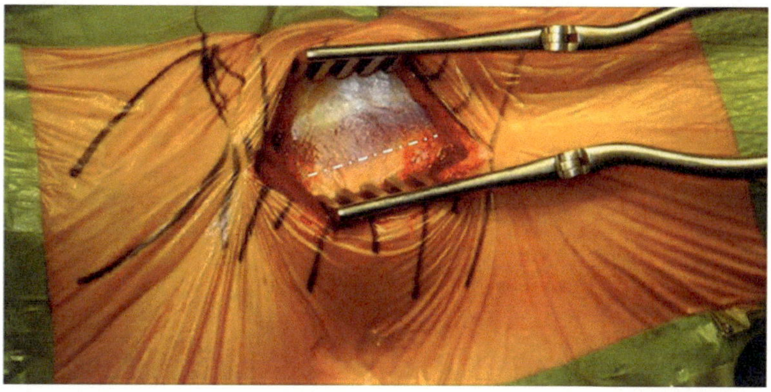

Figure 2.
Following the superficial dissection, the rectus femoris is visible. The deep layer of the dissection beneath the rectus is accessed by making a facial incision at the red-yellow junction (dotted white line) and retracting the rectus muscle belly medially (Right hip).

After retracting both the TFL and the rectus femoris muscle belly, the reflected head of the rectus (pars reflecta) can be seen inserting proximally on the anterior acetabulum (**Figure 3**). There is typically a fat pad with a small vessel at the insertion site. In cases where the pars reflecta is going to be released to allow the rectus femoris to relax and enhance surgical exposure, the fat pad needs to be resected and the vessel cauterized. *We recommend releasing the pars reflecta in all cases early on in the learning curve.* Carefully dissect the investing fascia over the rectus femoris to retract the rectus medially and expose the lateral femoral circumflex vessels (**Figure 4**). Once identified, these vessels need to be tied-off or thoroughly coagulated; electrocautery alone is typically not adequate.

After appropriately addressing the circumflex vessels, the peri-capsular fat is removed and the anterior hip capsule is exposed. While most surgeons are familiar with posterior capsular exposure, the anterior capsule creates a bare triangle between the iliocapsularis muscle medially, the gluteus medius laterally and the vastus lateralus distally. At this point, the option is to perform a capsulotomy (author's preferred technique) or a capsulectomy (**Figure 5**).

In addition to strong foundation of anatomy and surgical technique the use of retractors with appropriate placement is paramount for exposure and safety during the procedure. During acetabular exposure and preparation, the principal author utilizes two, 45 degree, pointed homan retractors for capsular exposure, placing one retractor inferior femoral neck space between the capsule and the muscle and the other retractor over the superior femoral neck protecting the gluteus medius muscle. Both retractors should be extracapsular; following capsulotomy, the retractors should be repositioned intracapsular. Additionally, a charnley retractor is used for hands free acetabular exposure. For right sided procedure, the anterior blade should be placed in the 1 o'clock position and the posterior blade in the 7 o'clock position. For femoral exposure, the use of a dark and stormy retractor placed over the posterior femoral neck, distal to the obturator externus muscle to elevate the femur for broaching.

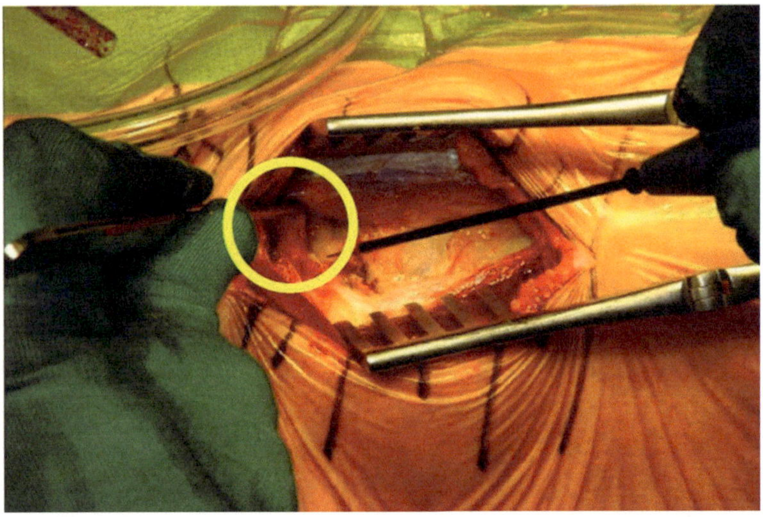

Figure 3.
The yellow circle denotes the pars reflects tendon as it originates from the anterior lip of the acetabulum (Right hip).

DOI: http://dx.doi.org/10.5772/intechopen.104398

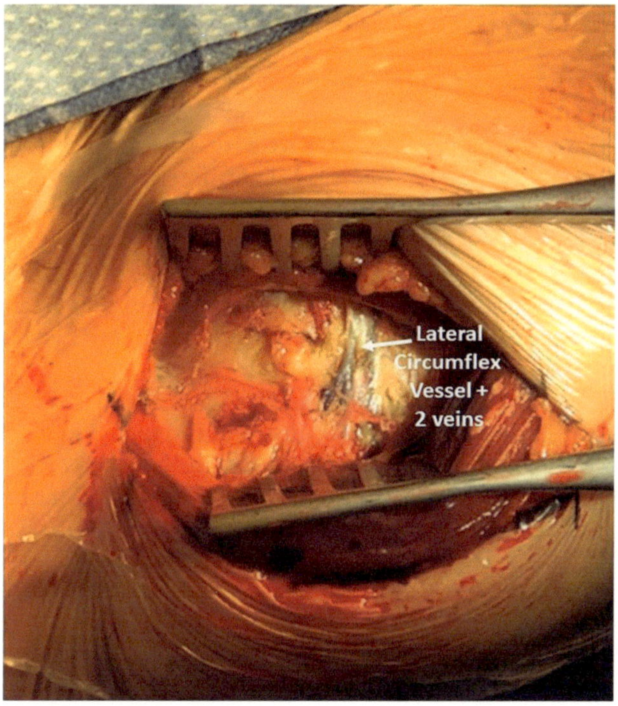

Figure 4.
The lateral circumflex vessels are typically visible just proximal to the vastus lateralis and course proximal lateral to distal medial. The artery typically courses with two accompanying venae comitantes (Right hip).

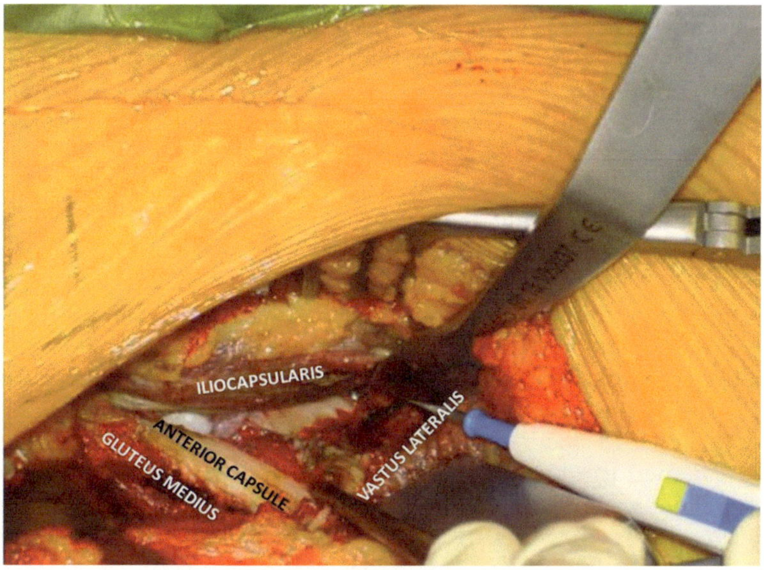

Figure 5.
The bare area in the anterior hip capsule is bordered by these muscles. This image shows the femoral head and neck after a triangular anterior capsulotomy has been performed (Right hip).

3. Methodological transition

The decision to transition from an alternative surgical approach is not one to take lightly. A surgeon must acknowledge that although they may have significant experience with performing a THA from an alternate surgical approach, the DAA THA is an entirely different procedure, especially if transitioning from a posterior approach – the anterior approach is oriented 90 degrees from your normal surgical view. Several reports highlight the dangers of inadequate preparation/planning for surgeons starting to perform the DAA leading to significantly increased surgical times and higher intra/post-operative complications [14]. Therefore, any surgeon deciding to take this step should create a comprehensive and thorough plan involving self-learning, mentorship, and cadaver sessions.

Once the decision to transition to the DAA has been made, and familiarization with the anatomy and surgical steps has been completed, the focus should be on proper surgical indications, common pitfalls, and understanding why you may struggle with portions of the procedure. E-learning (technique guides, digital modeling, online tutorials, surgical videos) has emerged as a powerful tool with many diverse teaching modalities, 24/7 access, and real-time measures progress through testing [15].

Surgical mentorship has been a pivotal aspect of training, emphasized by the Halstedian model of educating new surgeons [16]. Identifying a mentor is critical and it should be someone that is equally invested in you [17]. Observation of the surgical technique should be accompanied by creating a detailed, annotated surgical technique guide. This is the most critical part of making the transition and decreasing the learning curve. Similar to the sequence of surgical steps, the process of creating this surgical technique guide requires patience, diligence, and attention to detail. Additionally, this document should be used to acquaint the surgical team with the procedure, so they too can participate in minimizing the learning curve.

After an extensive observership and creating of a technique guide, hands-on cadaveric training is the next step in the sequence. The senior author assisted his mentor in the lab during a cadaveric demonstration of the procedure. Following the demonstration, the senior author performed a DAA THA on the contralateral hip with the assistance of his mentor. This cadaveric workshop helped to translate what was seen in the operating room during observation into the tangible ability of performing the procedure prior to going live on an actual patient.

After selectively identifying patients that should be considered candidates for a DAA THA (**Table 1**), reverse surgical observation by the mentor was arranged. The first two DAA THAs were observed by the mentor with real-time feedback and guidance provided during the operation. This portion of the training significantly decreased the anxiety associated with performing a DAA for the first time. The mentor should help with identifying your tendencies and anticipating difficulties (e.g. improper retractor placement or limb positioning) before they arise.

All team members should be a part of the learning process. This is not limited to the surgical team performing the procedure (surgeon, Fellow/Resident, advanced practice provider) but should include the scrub technician, circulating nurse, radiology technician, and the anesthesia team. A pre-operative planning session with the entire team can be very helpful early on in the learning curve. More importantly, a post-operative debrief after every case should be conducted with the team to determine what went well, what didn't go well, what did we learn, and what should we should do differently for the next case. This process allows for iterative improvements with performing the DAA safely and reproducibly.

Indications	Contraindications
Non-muscular patients	Muscular patients
Thin patients	Obese patients
Patients with normal bone quality	Patients with osteoporosis
Long valgus femoral necks	Short varus femoral necks
Narrow iliac flares	Wide iliac flares
Dorr Type B femoral canal	Dorr Type A femoral canal
	Retained hardware
	Severe dysplasia
	Proximal femoral deformity

Table 1.
Indications and contraindications to guide patient selection during the learning curve.

4. Continued learning

Creating a schedule that allows for continued learning is imperative. The senior author re-visited his mentor after case #30; the surgical team was included as a part of this visitation. After 60 cases, the senior author arranged for repeat reverse visitation by the mentor to observe and identify any additional tweaks in the technique that should be incorporated. Lastly, data collection is helpful to monitor your tendencies and refine the technique to recognize additional efficiencies.

5. Conclusion

It is important to stress that although you may be a skilled arthroplasty surgeon and experienced in other THA approaches, learning the DAA approach is like starting from scratch. Creating a comprehensive, and methodological, training plan is crucial to achieving clinical success while maintain the safety of your patients. Embracing the significance of self-learning and critique, active mentorship, and substantial hands-on training will maximize your time spent re-training. It is important to understand that once the training period is complete, the learning period continues. Finally, it is imperative to incorporate every member of the operative team as each member plays a critical role in executing the procedure and thus achieving a favorable clinical outcome. In conclusion, transitioning to the direct anterior approach is not a spectator sport – this approach requires dedication, diligence, attention to detail, and patience!

Author details

Bijan Dehghani[1*], Avi Dravid[2], Praneeth Thota[2] and Neil P. Sheth[3]

1 Orthopaedic Surgery Resident, University of Pennsylvania, Philadelphia, PA

2 University of Pennsylvania, Philadelphia, PA

3 Chief of Orthopaedic Surgery – Pennsylvania Hospital, Associate Professor of Orthopaedic Surgery, University of Pennsylvania, Philadelphia, PA

*Address all correspondence to: bijan.dehghani@pennmedicine.upenn.edu

References

[1] Aumiller W, Kleuser T. Trends in total hip arthroplasty. Journal of the American Academy of Physician Assistants. 2019;**32**(3):51-53. DOI: 10.1097/01.JAA.0000553394.43873.76

[2] Moretti VM, Post ZD. Surgical approaches for total hip arthroplasty. Indian Journal of Orthopaedics. 2017;**51**(4):368-376. DOI: 10.4103/ortho.IJOrtho_317_16

[3] Sloan M, Premkumar A, Sheth N. Projected volume of primary total joint arthroplasty in the U.S., 2014 to 2030. The Journal of Bone and Joint Surgery. 2018;**100**(17):1455-1460. DOI: 10.2106/JBJS.17.01617

[4] Singh JA, Yu S, Lang C, Cleveland J. Rates of total joint replacement in the United States: Future projections to 2020-2040 using the national inpatient sample. The Journal of Rheumatology. 2019;**46**(9):1134-1140. DOI: 10.3899/jrheum.170990

[5] Rachbauer F, Kain MS, Leunig M. The history of the anterior approach to the hip. Orthopedic Clinics of North America. 2009;**40**(3):311-320. DOI: 10.1016/j.ocl.2009.02.007

[6] Kong L, Chen L, Sun L, Tian X. Direct anterior approach or posterior approach in total hip arthroplasty: A direct comparative study protocol. Medicine (Baltimore). 2020;**99**(42):e22717. DOI: 10.1097/MD.0000000000022717

[7] Higgins BT, Barlow DR, Heagerty NE, Lin TJ. Anterior vs. posterior approach for total hip arthroplasty, a systematic review and meta-analysis. Journal of Arthroplasty. 2015;**30**(3):419-434. DOI: 10.1016/j.arth.2014.10.020

[8] Barrett WP, Turner SE, Leopold JP. Prospective randomized study of direct anterior vs postero-lateral approach for total hip arthroplasty. Journal of Arthroplasty. 2013;**28**(9):1634-1638. DOI: 10.1016/j.arth.2013.01.034

[9] Wang Z, Bao H, Hou J. Direct anterior versus lateral approaches for clinical outcomes after total hip arthroplasty: A meta-analysis. Journal of Orthopaedic Surgery and Research. 2019;**14**(63). DOI: 10.1186/s13018-019-1095-z

[10] Martin CT, Pugely AJ, Gao Y, Clark CR. A comparison of hospital length of stay and short-term morbidity between the anterior and the posterior approaches to total hip arthroplasty. Journal of Arthroplasty. 2013;**28**(5):849-854. DOI: 10.1016/j.arth.2012.10.029

[11] Boe R, Sheth NP, et al. Soft-tissue balancing in total hip arthroplasty. JBJS Reviews. 2021;**9**(2):e20.0016. DOI: 10.2106/JBJS.RVW.20.00116

[12] Martin JR, Nikolaus OB, Springer BD. Direct anterior total hip arthroplasty: Solicitation and industry. Annals of Joints. 2018;**3**(54). DOI: 10.21037/aoj.2018.05.07

[13] Nairn L, Gyemi L, Gouveia K, Ekhtiari S, Khanna V. The learning curve for the direct anterior total hip arthroplasty: A systematic review. International Orthopaetics. 2021;**45**(8):1971-1982. DOI: 10.1007/s00264-021-04986-7

[14] Pirruccio K, Evangelista PJ, Haw J, Goldberg T, Sheth NP. Safely implementing the direct anterior total hip arthroplasty: A methodological approach to minimizing the learning curve. Journal of the American

Academy of Orthopaedic Surgeons. 2020;**28**(22):930-936. DOI: 10.5435/JAAOS-D-19-00752

[15] Tarpada SP, Morris MT, Burton DA. E-learning in orthopedic surgery training: A systematic review. Journal of Orthopaetics. 2016;**13**(4):425-430. DOI: 10.1016/j.jor.2016.09.004

[16] Assael LA. Every surgeon needs mentors: A Halsteadian/Socratic model in the modern age. Journal of Oral and Maxillofacial Surgery. 2010;**68**(6):1217-1218. DOI: 10.1016/j.joms.2010.04.005

[17] Entezami P, Franzblau LE, Chung KC. Mentorship in surgical training: A systematic review. Hand (N Y). 2012;**7**(1):30-36. DOI: 10.1007/s11552-011-9379-8